SEGRETI DEL BIOHACKING

Le Vere Tecniche per Aumentare Salute,
Longevità, Stile di Vita, Costruire Abitudini
Sane e Crescita di Massa Muscolare.

Giovanni Sacco

SOMMARIO

INTRODUZIONE

Questo libro è stato scritto con l'intenzione di aiutare le persone che vogliono in un modo o nell'altro, migliorare la qualità della vita. Introdurremo il metodo del biohacking, usato da molti personaggi famosi, giocatori dell'NBA, lottatori dell'UFC, atleti delle Olimpiadi, imprenditori milionari e miliardari della Silicon Valley. Viene usato per aumentare prestazioni fisiche e mentali, distruggere ansia, attacchi di panico e nevrosi.

Anche Bill Gates ha detto che, se fosse oggi un ragazzo, applicherebbe senza dubbio il biohacking.

In questo libro non vi parlerò del fatto che dovrete calmarvi, essere meno stressati ecc. Vi darò una risposta concreta e giusta su quali pratiche dover applicare per una vita migliore.

Se ti trovi di fronte a sintomi come paura improvvisa della morte, attacchi d'ansia accompagnati dall'incapacità di pensare chiaramente, perdita di coscienza, eccitazione e aumento dell'aggressività, ansia, preoccupazione e paura, allora questo libro fa per voi! Vedremo come gli effetti della temperatura possono essere benefici sul corpo e sull'organismo. Vi darò una risposta su come hackerare i famosi mitocondri, che sono la base della fonte di energia che il nostro corpo ha. Anche se avrete affrontato terapie che si discostano dalla medicina tradizionale, ed esse sono state inutili, non preoccupatevi. Sono sicuro che il biohacking vi potrà aiutare come non mai. Basterà applicare quanto scritto in questo libro, senza paura e ansia.

Quindi, se stai cercando serenità, una vita migliore, migliori prestazioni mentali e fisiche, aumento della massa muscolare e uno stile di vita più sano… che aspetti! Inizia subito a leggere questo libro e queste fantastiche e preziose informazioni. Buona lettura.

Se questo libro vi piacerà, sarò molto contento sapere cosa avrai apprezzato di più attraverso una piccola recensione direttamente su Amazon. Grazie!

Capitolo 1

INTRODUZIONE AL BIOHACKING

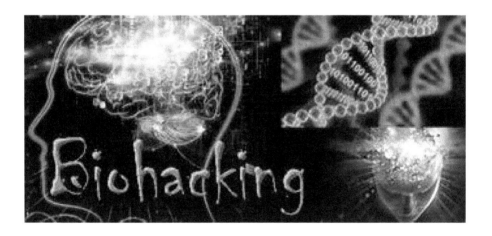

Chi è un Biohacker?

Un **biohacker** è una persona che massimizza il suo potenziale biologico attraverso vari mezzi e tecniche. Tutto ciò che migliora la tua biologia fa parte del biohacking.

Per esempio:

- Rafforzare il corpo attraverso gli allenamenti (i muscoli sono una parte della tua biologia, quindi massimizzare la forza, la resistenza o le dimensioni è un aumento del potenziale biologico).

- Pelle resistente al sole (se prendi il sole per diverse settimane in giorni di buon sole e hai una pelle di colore scuro, allora questo è biohacking, perché il suo potenziale protettivo è aumentato).

- Anche l'ottimizzazione della nutrizione fa parte del biohacking, perché eliminando i prodotti nocivi e aggiungendo prodotti sani, si può migliorare significativamente sia la biologia degli organi interni che l'aspetto, insieme alla produttività.

- Amplificazione dovuta agli effetti della temperatura. Il livello dosato di stress da temperatura stimola il nostro corpo, migliorando molto il nostro potenziale biologico.

- Rafforzamento attraverso la meditazione e pratiche simili. Dove va la coscienza, va anche il corpo. La meditazione è il modo migliore per calmare i pensieri.

• Prendere integratori e stimolanti. Esiste anche questa opzione per migliorare il tuo corpo/mente. Inoltre, molti integratori (come l'Omega 3) sono davvero importanti. Ma il più delle volte, il valore di questo metodo, è notevolmente esagerato.

Il BIOHAKING è l'attività volta a massimizzare il tuo potenziale biologico. Questo include anche il lavoro del tuo cervello, perché è completamente dipendente dalla nostra biologia. Il cervello e la coscienza non possono vivere senza un corpo. I BIOHAKES sono metodi e tecniche specifiche per aumentare il proprio potenziale biologico.

Per esempio, quando state migliorando la termoregolazione del vostro corpo con una sauna o un allenamento, si tratta di biohacking. Senza una corretta amministrazione del nostro corpo, lo stress può essere troppo alto e distruggerlo, invece di rafforzarlo.

Hack Temperatura

Di cosa tratta questa sezione? Questo materiale riguarda il biohacking usando lo stress da temperatura dosata sul nostro corpo. Arriverai a sapere come usare la corretta somministrazione di alte e basse temperature per migliorare i parametri biologici e neurologici del tuo cervello e del sistema nervoso. Il numero di miglioramenti che puoi ottenere usando le tecniche descritte è molto ampio.

- **Neurogenesi**. È l'innovamento dei neuroni del cervello usando la bassa temperatura, la proteina dello shock freddo. Miglioramento delle funzioni cerebrali, della memoria e dell'intelligenza.

- **Biogenesi**. È il rinnovamento e aumento del numero di mitocondri delle "stazioni energetiche del corpo". Migliora il tono del corpo e l'energia.

- **Miglioramento passivo dell'ossidazione dei grassi**. Con l'aiuto degli effetti della temperatura, è possibile cambiare la proporzione di grasso bianco (energia) / marrone (calore). Così, è possibile aumentare la combustione passiva dei grassi del 90-350%

- **Sintesi proteica e rilascio di GH**. Le alte temperature aumentano la sintesi proteica del 30%, e il rilascio di GH aumenta di 2 volte. In alcuni esperimenti, c'è stato un aumento di 5 volte. Il tutto senza alcun farmaco o droga.

Il GH è conosciuto anche come ormone della crescita, ed è prodotto dall'ipofisi. Durante l'adolescenza, i livelli di GH aumentano notevolmente, stimolando la crescita della statura, aumentando la ritenzione di azoto e favorendo l'ossidazione delle scorte lipidiche.

- **Rafforzamento del sistema cardiovascolare**. Gli effetti della temperatura restringono e dilatano i nostri vasi sanguigni. Tale formazione migliora la loro condizione e funzionalità.

▪ **Protezione del collagene**. Usando le basse temperature, possiamo bloccare il catabolismo del collagene nel nostro corpo. Questo significa articolazioni sane e pelle elastica

▪ **Rafforzamento dell'immunità**. Si è notato da tempo che i nuotatori del nord quasi non si ammalano. Il fatto è che le basse temperature aumentano significativamente il numero di cellule immunitarie.

Il materiale è composto da 3 sezioni, ovvero "osmosi con basse temperature", "osmosi con alte temperature" e "Schemi di somministrazione per diversi compiti".

Cos'è l'osmosi?

L'osmosi è l'effetto stimolante di dosi moderate di stress sui sistemi del corpo. A metà del secolo scorso, alcuni scienziati hanno scoperto che lo stress moderato (bassa temperatura, alta temperatura, ipossia, attività fisica, fame, ecc.) ha un effetto stimolante su vari sistemi del corpo. In altre parole, il nostro corpo ha bisogno di uno stress moderato per un funzionamento normale.

In questo caso, si verifica un effetto stimolante e un miglioramento del potenziale biologico. ogni persona è una sorta di "sistema interno" di organi e processi che interagisce con il sistema esterno (il mondo). Lo stato ideale a cui ogni sistema aspira è uno stato di equilibrio. Se non c'è equilibrio, e il sistema esterno è "più forte", allora si verifica la distruzione dei sistemi interni.

Per esempio, se il corpo brucia in un incendio allora è un male per il nostro corpo. D'altra parte, se il corpo non prende mai il sole, allora si indebolisce a causa della mancanza di vitamina D. Tutto ha bisogno di equilibrio. Tutti gli animali del nostro pianeta sono programmati per risolvere problemi di sopravvivenza biologica, uno dei quali è il risparmio energetico. E lo stato energeticamente più favorevole di qualsiasi organismo è uno stato di equilibrio con l'ambiente. In questo stato, l'organismo è produttivo e si sente bene perché consuma poca energia. Con lo sviluppo della tecnologia, l'umanità ha imparato a ridurre artificialmente l'impatto dell'ambiente esterno.

Abbiamo inventato vestiti, case e riscaldamento per non congelare. Abbiamo inventato macchine e meccanismi per muoverci meno e sforzarci. Abbiamo creato una tecnologia alimentare che rende facile ottenere energia in eccesso da cibi economici. Di fatto, nella ricerca del comfort, abbiamo finalmente **disturbato l'equilibrio** tra l'uomo e l'ambiente. Pensateci: abbiamo tecnologie mediche e medicine uniche, ma questo non aiuta a ridurre il numero di persone malate. Ogni anno ce ne sono sempre di più. Cose come malattie cardiovascolari, infarti, ictus, cancro, diabete, obesità, ecc. Da dove vengono? A causa di uno squilibrio.

Per esempio, se una persona mangia ogni giorno cibi dolci e grassi, questo porta al diabete, alle malattie cardiache e al cancro, perché si ottiene ma non si spende. In questo modo l'equilibrio è disturbato e questo porta alla distruzione del corpo. L'osmosi è un modo per ripristinare lo stato di equilibrio del corpo e dell'ambiente. Questo avviene grazie all'effetto stimolante di dosi moderate di stress. Il tuo corpo riceve esattamente la dose di stress che lo stimola ad aumentare il potenziale biologico.

Quanto è pericoloso il biohacking?

In questo materiale parleremo del biohacking usando l'osmosi della temperatura (impatto delle alte o basse temperature) e non solo.

Le temperature alte o basse possono essere pericolose? Sicuramente sì. La questione è il volume e la durata dello stress da temperatura. Tutto è veleno e tutto è medicina, come diceva il vecchio proverbio. La differenza è solo nel dosaggio. Per ottenere un effetto stimolante, è necessario che lo stress sia sufficiente e in nessun caso non sia eccessivo. Ecco la differenza:

- **Stress sufficiente** = l'organismo può adattarsi ad esso (effetto stimolante)

- **Stress eccessivo** = l'organismo non può adattarsi (troppo, distruzione)

Per esempio, uno stress a bassa temperatura sufficiente stimola la neurogenesi, la biogenesi, l'immunità, la combustione dei grassi, ecc. Tuttavia, se lo stress a bassa temperatura è troppo grande o troppo a lungo (stress eccessivo), allora ci verrà la polmonite. Nel primo caso, otteniamo un aumento nel corpo. E nel secondo caso, distruggiamo il corpo con gli stessi strumenti. Se fate tutto gradualmente e nell'ambito dello schema di somministrazione che vi darò, allora tutto andrà. Avremo abbastanza stress, non un eccesso.

Osmosi con le Basse Temperature

Lo stress a bassa temperatura a breve termine stimola un aumento del potenziale biologico di vari organi e sistemi del corpo. Avrai notato che dopo l'immersione in acqua fredda, ti senti molto meglio e il tuo cervello si libera. Vi è familiare? Questo è un effetto tipico dello stress da bassa temperatura. All'inizio si sente disagio, o addirittura sofferenza a causa del freddo, e dopo si sente l'aumento di tutti i sistemi del corpo. Anche un solo stress da bassa temperatura stimola vari sistemi e organi del nostro corpo, migliorando il potenziale biologico. Tuttavia, se cominci a "coccolare" REGOLARMENTE il tuo corpo con stress a bassa temperatura, allora cominciano ad accadere cose veramente fantastiche.

Diventi un superuomo, in un certo senso. La tua mente, la resistenza, l'aspetto (il grasso brucia), il sistema cardiovascolare, lo stato delle articolazioni e dei legamenti e l'immunità cambiano. Ma lasciate che vi parli di tutte le "chicche" in ordine.

Brucia grassi

Ti piacerebbe mangiare di più è perdere peso più facilmente? Immaginate che questa cosa non richiede nemmeno esercizi estenuanti. Sembra una favola? Tuttavia, questo è esattamente ciò che accade grazie alla "termogenesi fredda". Lo stress regolare a bassa temperatura cambia la proporzione di grasso bianco / marrone nel corpo e quindi aumenta il trasferimento di calore e il metabolismo del 90-350%. Tutti i mammiferi, a differenza di quelli a sangue freddo, mantengono una temperatura corporea costante dissipando l'energia termica dalle riserve di grasso. Questo è necessario per la sopravvivenza nei climi freddi. Il grasso non è solo una fonte di energia, ma anche una fonte di calore se fa freddo. Il problema è che per tutta la vita viviamo in condizioni troppo confortevoli (senza freddo) e quindi non usiamo il meccanismo di spendere il grasso per aumentare la temperatura. Se il tuo corpo è colpito da una bassa temperatura, allora reagisci in questi modi. **Rabbrividisci**, e il freddo fa contrarre rapidamente i muscoli per convertire l'energia meccanica in calore. Questo si esprime nel tremore del tuo corpo. **Non rabbrividisci**. Il freddo coinvolge la termogenesi bruciando il grasso marrone e una speciale proteina della membrana mitocondriale interna chiamata *"Termogenina"*.

Il procedimento è questo → Stress da bassa temperatura → Rilascio di noradrenalina in risposta allo stress → La noradrenalina stimola le goccioline di grasso nelle cellule di grasso marrone → Attiva la proteina Termogenina → La Termogenina "scioglie" la conduttività della membrana. → Termogenesi fredda (i grassi vengono spesi per riscaldare il corpo).

Osmosi con le Alte Temperature

Lo stress a breve termine ad alta temperatura stimola specificamente un aumento del potenziale biologico di vari organi e sistemi del corpo. Uno dei fattori più importanti che influenzano il potenziale biologico del tuo corpo sono i "Mitocondri". La tua salute, il tuo benessere e la tua energia dipendono completamente dallo stato dei mitocondri. Vari effetti della temperatura hanno una forte influenza sia sul lavoro dei mitocondri, che sul loro numero. Ma andiamo con ordine.

Mitocondri, "stazioni di energia"

I mitocondri sono il generatore di energia del tuo corpo. La sua funzione principale è l'ossidazione dei composti organici e l'utilizzo dell'energia rilasciata durante il loro decadimento per generare potenziale elettrico, sintesi di ATP e termogenesi.

L'ATP è chiamata anche con il nome di "Adenosina trifosfato", che è una molecola costituita da adenosina e da tre gruppi fosfato. Serve per fornire alla cellula l'energia necessaria per svolgere qualsiasi tipo di lavoro biologico

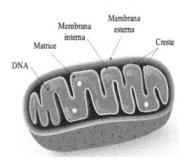

MITOCONDRIO

Tutti i nostri organi e sistemi corporei sono completamente dipendenti dai mitocondri, perché tutti possono funzionare solo grazie all'energia che riceviamo dall'ambiente esterno. Ogni essere vivente ha bisogno di cibo. Per quale motivo? Per produrre l'energia necessaria alla vita. Se una persona non riceve cibo per molto tempo, allora questo alla fine porta alla morte perché non c'è abbastanza energia per la vita. In generale, il cibo che mangiamo viene trasformato in energia e ciò avviene nei mitocondri.

L'essenza dei mitocondri è prendere elettroni da grassi e carboidrati. Questo processo è chiamato "fosforilazione ossidativa". Durante questo processo, l'energia è generata come risultato dell'ossidazione dei nutrienti (prevalentemente carboidrati e grassi). La fosforilazione ossidativa è un metabolismo in cui l'energia generata, durante l'ossidazione dei nutrienti, viene immagazzinata nei mitocondri delle cellule sotto forma di ATP. L'ATP, come detto, è l'unità energetica di base del nostro corpo. Ecco perché, a scuola, ci siamo abituati al fatto che i mitocondri sono la "stazione energetica" delle nostre cellule. Se i mitocondri funzionano male, allora questo porta quasi sempre a malattie croniche associate a un metabolismo intracellulare alterato.

Un esempio classico è il cancro. Spesso si sente dire che il cancro è una malattia genetica. Tuttavia, fortunatamente questo non è del tutto vero. Il più delle volte, i tumori mutano sotto l'influenza di disturbi metabolici, e non a causa della "cattiva genetica". Pertanto, nella maggior parte dei casi, possiamo dire che il cancro è un problema metabolico, non genetico. Ho parlato con ottimi medici specializzati in oncologia e mi è stato detto: c'è una chiara correlazione tra il metabolismo dei carboidrati e il cancro. Chiunque mangi carboidrati e dolci in eccesso ha una resistenza all'insulina e una maggiore possibilità di ammalarsi di cancro. Bene, dato che stiamo parlando di metabolismo, questo significa sempre che abbiamo a che fare con i mitocondri in un modo o nell'altro. Perché il nostro metabolismo con l'ambiente avviene in gran parte attraverso i mitocondri. Purtroppo, nei paesi sviluppati, una persona su 2 dopo i 40 anni ha acquisito una disfunzione mitocondriale. Questo si esprime nel fatto che la quantità e/o la produttività del lavoro delle "stazioni energetiche" è ridotta.

La situazione è assolutamente tipica e si può facilmente trovare un'analogia nella vita quotidiana. Ricordate il vostro precedente telefono? La sua batteria era sufficiente per tutto il giorno quando era nuovo. Tuttavia, dopo sei mesi, notate che dovete ricaricare più volte il telefono durante il giorno. Se continuate l'uso attivo del dispositivo, allora arriverete al punto che andrete ovunque con un caricatore perché la batteria del telefono diventerà sempre peggiore per mantenere la carica. Ad un certo punto, o si cambia la batteria o si compra un nuovo telefono. Sfortunatamente, la gente non ha ancora imparato a cambiare il proprio corpo con uno più giovane. Pertanto, otteniamo la stessa serie di problemi associati all'invecchiamento delle nostre "batterie" come i nostri dispositivi portatili.

Ma dov'è il biohacking? Qual è la connessione? Proprio in questo luogo il BIOHAKING sta diventando rilevante. Perché il biohacking è un miglioramento del tuo potenziale biologico e i nostri mitocondri sono i motori chiave di esso. Se sei pieno di energia e forza, allora questo è grazie ai tuoi mitocondri. In questo caso, è ovvio che il tuo potenziale biologico è alto.

In seguito, vedremo tutti i consigli pratici.

L'Hacking dei Mitocondri

L'energia: senza energia le cellule muoiono. Le cellule, a differenza di come si dice, non vengono nutrite da carboidrati, proteine ecc., ma la fonte di energia è l'ATP (adenosina trifosfato). L'ATP viene prodotta dai mitocondri. Come già detto, i mitocondri sono organelli cellulari e sono considerati la centrale energetica della cellula. Al loro interno avviene la respirazione cellulare, con cui sono in grado di produrre grandi quantità di energia sotto forma di molecole di ATP.

Quindi sono contenuti nelle nostre cellule e sono responsabili della produzione dell'energia.
L'ATP Sintasi è il vero carburante energetico delle nostre cellule.

Il mitocondrio ha la forma di un fagiolo e si riproducono in modo indipendente.
I mitocondri sono contenuti in tutto il corpo con maggioranza nel cervello, cuore, occhi, ovaie (donne), testicoli (uomini – sono responsabili della produzione de testosterone).

Salute dei mitocondri

Alla base dell'invecchiamento, c'è il deterioramento dei mitocondri. Si stima che tra i 30 e i 60 anni i mitocondri perdano il 50% dell'efficienza. Seguendo i consigli dati, i mitocondri si possono mantenere in salute ed efficienti per tutta la vita, "hackerandoli" nel modo giusto. Se i mitocondri funzionano bene, producono più energia e di conseguenza funziona meglio l'organismo.

Quindi se vogliamo hackerare la nostra biologia dobbiamo hackerare i mitocondri

Come si hackerano i mitocondri?

Per hackerare i mitocondri bisogna:

- Miglior alimentazione possibile (vedremo dopo gli alimenti).
- Ossigenoterapia con esercizi fisici appropriati e miglioramento della circolazione sanguigna. È risaputa l'importanza dell'ambiente in cui si vive e dell'aria che respiriamo).
- Stabilizzazione dei livelli di zucchero nel sangue.
- Ottimizzazione dei livelli ormonali. Gli ormoni sono importanti in quanto governano ogni aspetto della nostra biologia.
- Depurazione efficace ed eliminazione delle tossine. Già si sapeva che le tossine sono negative sul nostro organismo. Ora sappiamo che danneggiano anche i mitocondri.
- Quantità funzionali di stress che innescano l'autofagia e l'apoptosi.
L'autofagia è un processo importante che avviene all'interno delle cellule dove quest'ultime distruggono il materiale danneggiato e lo utilizzano a scopo energetico. Avviene una pulizia dove le cellule diventano più efficienti e in salute. L'apoptosi è un processo che riguarda la morte programmata delle cellule. È un meccanismo naturale e spesso un'anomalia in esso è causa di diverse patologie (tipo cancro).
- Allenamento adeguato digiuno ben organizzato.
- Esposizione alla luce di migliore qualità ed eliminazione di quella cattiva.
- Integrazione di sostanze chiave. L'integrazione giusta può dare una sferzata di energia ai mitocondri.
- Esposizione a determinati ambienti in determinate modalità, che danno il via a numerose reazioni positive per l'intero organismo.

Biohacking e Ormoni

Gli ormoni sono la chiave per un corpo e una mente top

Cosa sono gli ormoni?

Gli ormoni sono dei messaggeri chimici che sono prodotti da alcune ghiandole (dette ghiandole endocrine in quanto versano gli ormoni direttamente nel sangue, a differenza di quelle esocrine che il contenuto lo espellono fuori dal corpo, come le ghiandole sudoripare con il sudore). Vengono rilasciati nel sangue e questi raggiungeranno particolari cellule e organi bersaglio (è una comunicazione chimica, che è più lenta rispetto alla comunicazione nervosa).

Ogni ghiandola produce ormoni con diversi scopi (chi controlla il metabolismo, chi per le donne la crescita del seno e latte, chi la funzione sessuale, chi controlla la funzione ed umore conoscitivi, chi il mantenimento della temperatura corporea e della sete ecc.).

Le principali ghiandole endocrine sono la Ghiandola Pineale, Ipofisi, Tiroide, Timo, Ghiandole surrenali, Pancreas, Ovario (femmine), Testicoli (maschile).

Gli ormoni, in campo Biohacking, sono molto importanti, soprattutto quelli "tiroidei" (T3, T4) e "steroidei" (testosterone). Quindi, gli ormoni sono un aspetto su cui il biohacker si deve concentrare per hackerare prestazioni fisiche e mentali. Essendo messaggeri nell'organismo, gli ormoni possono di conseguenza mandare messaggi con influenza positiva e negativa. L'hackeraggio del sistema ormonale è fondamentale nel biohacking (con le pratiche suggerite andremo a incentivare la produzione ormonale positiva in modo da raggiungere prestazioni fisiche/mentali ottime).

Capitolo 2

MIGLIORAMENTO GENERALE DELLA SALUTE CON LA TEMPERATURA

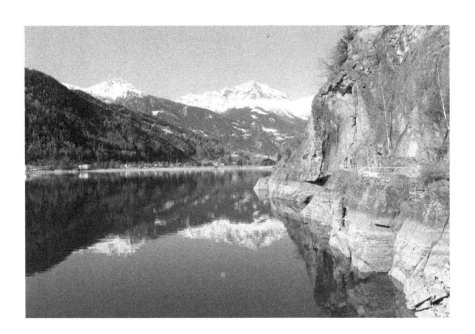

Con l'età, le persone cominciano ad ammalarsi sempre di più. Di regola, in questo momento inizia la ricerca di "pillole magiche" per curare un organismo. Una tale "pillola" stranamente esiste. Si tratta di uno stress regolare ad alta temperatura. Ci sono esperimenti che mostrano una riduzione del 33-77% del dolore di artrite e reumatismi con l'uso regolare della sauna. Inoltre, l'effetto ottenuto è stato mantenuto per 6 mesi dopo la cessazione degli effetti dell'alta temperatura. Nel 2015, gli scienziati americani hanno studiato la dipendenza del bagno turco e le malattie cardiovascolari. Hanno concluso che c'è un chiaro effetto inverso: più sauna o bagno turco, meno malattie cardiovascolari e migliore salute.

Sauna

In particolare, una delle osservazioni è stata fatta dalla American Medical Association. Si tratta di una ricerca molto interessante perché 2.300 uomini vi hanno partecipato per 20 anni. Gli scienziati hanno scoperto che uomini che facevano saune, avevano meno malattie cardiovascolari. Per esempio: 2-3 volte a settimana si avrà il 27% di riduzione del rischio di malattie cardiovascolari. 4-7 volte a settimana si avrà il 50% di riduzione di queste malattie e un 66% di riduzione del rischio di demenza, Alzheimer e mortalità.

Casi in cui è pericolosa la sauna

Ci sono diverse situazioni in cui non è necessario andare in sauna, ad esempio:

- Se sei una donna incinta.

- Se sei un uomo che pensa di fare un bambino (l'alta temperatura influenza la qualità e la mobilità dello sperma).

- Se la testa non è protetta (usare un cappuccio alle alte temperature).

- Se sei ubriaco (l'alcol è un diuretico da solo).

- Se si è disidratati (è necessario bere acqua prima e dopo la sauna per compensare la perdita).

Come Migliorare Costantemente gli Effetti sul Corpo?

Affinché l'osmosi abbia un effetto positivo sul tuo corpo, le pratiche devono essere eseguite CONSAPEVOLMENTE. Se le procedure ti causano solo emozioni negative, allora devi ridurre il livello di stress, o cambiare il focus del tuo pensiero (trovare cose positive in quello che sta succedendo).

Prima di esporre il tuo corpo allo stress termico, devi prima curarlo completamente da eventuali malattie che hai, altrimenti, i "focolai di malattia" possono crescere e la vostra condizione peggiorerà. Se hai processi infiammatori nel corpo (appendici, tonsille, denti, prostata, ecc.), allora devi prima curarli. Se hai problemi con il sistema cardiovascolare, è consigliabile consultare il tuo medico. Dovrete inoltre essere sistematici se volete beneficiare delle basse temperature. Questo vuol dire che dovrete esporvi regolarmente durante l'anno. Quindi, anche in estate, cerca di lavarti sotto una doccia fredda o fai una criosauna.

Affinché lo stress non sia troppo grande, è necessario aumentarlo gradualmente. Dovete passare costantemente da temperature più morbide a quelle più dure. Per esempio, si può iniziare con una passata con un asciugamano freddo o immergendo le mani/piedi in acqua fredda. Con la crescita dell'adattamento si può passare a una doccia fredda e poi all'immersione completa in vasche fredde. Altrimenti, il rischio di ottenere uno stress eccessivo (invece che sufficiente) è molto alto.

Per fare questo, è necessario utilizzare prima gli effetti "leggeri", e poi quelli più "pesanti". Se stiamo parlando di basse temperature, queste sono le fasi che di solito si fanno:

- **Spugnatura**. Questa è la procedura iniziale ed è la più morbida. Può essere applicata all'inizio, ed è adatta anche ai bambini. La linea di fondo è che si inzuppa asciugamano / spugna in acqua fredda, e poi costantemente pulire il petto, schiena, gambe, ecc. Infine asciugatevi con un panno asciutto.

- **Immersione parziale.** Riempire la vasca con acqua fredda. In primo luogo, immergere le mani e il viso. Dopo di che, mettete una bacinella sul pavimento e immergetevi le gambe. È utile lavare i piedi con acqua fredda durante tutto l'anno. Per prima cosa, puoi iniziare a fare queste immersioni con acqua a 25 C, e poi abbassare gradualmente il grado fino a 5-10 C. Per fare questo, ogni settimana puoi ridurre di 1 C la temperatura dell'acqua. Non avere fretta di fare tutto velocemente. Nessuno vi mette fretta. La regolarità è molto più importante del tasso di diminuzione della temperatura.

•**Doccia fredda**. Questo è il passo successivo nel tuo adattamento all'esposizione al freddo. Nelle fasi iniziali, entrate in una doccia fredda per 2-5 secondi. Molto velocemente. Man mano che ci si abitua, si noterà che si può stare più a lungo, e il piacere dopo la procedura diventa sempre più grande. Un'altra opzione è quella di iniziare con temperature confortevoli e gradualmente, nel corso di diversi mesi, ridurle a quelle di cui hai bisogno.

•**Immersione completa**. Questo è l'impatto più aggressivo di tutti. Si immerge completamente il corpo in acqua o in una massa d'aria fredda. Bisogna passare a questo stress solo dopo essersi adattati a impatti più morbidi.

Quando sei immerso in acqua fredda, la cosa più importante è preparare gradualmente il tuo corpo per questo. Assicurati di avere una persona che possa sostenerti. Non immergetevi mai da soli nella buca di ghiaccio. Ci dovrebbe essere sempre qualcuno nelle vicinanze. Inoltre, cercate laghi non profondi. Alla mia prima immersione, entrambe le mie gambe hanno avuto un crampo. Nell'acqua profonda, può essere pericoloso.

Come eseguire il raffreddamento per le persone principianti?

•**Spugnatura**. Si imbeve una spugna o un asciugamano in acqua fredda e poi si passa sulla parte superiore del corpo. Poi si fa con la parte inferiore. Dopo il passaggio della spugna è necessario asciugare il corpo con un asciugamano asciutto. Questo è il modo più delicato di impatto.

• **Doccia fredda e calda.** Bisogna passare prima al freddo, poi al caldo e così via. Girare il rubinetto prima nella posizione calda, che si può tollerare. Poi ruota la maniglia nella posizione fredda, che potrai tollerare 30-60 secondi.

• **Doccia fredda alla fine.** Le vostre docce dovrebbero terminare con acqua fredda. Mettere nella posizione più fredda, che potrai sopportare 60-120 secondi.

• **Vestiti leggeri in autunno/inverno.** Cerca di uscire con una maglietta leggera e pantaloncini. Riempi la vasca con acqua fredda e immergi le mani per 60 secondi. Immergere i piedi in acqua fredda per 60 secondi. Puoi prendere due bacinelle e riempirle con acqua diversa (fredda e calda). Immergi i piedi in una bacinella e le mani in un'altra. Dopo di che, scambia le posizioni.

• **Ghiaccio.** Mettete del ghiaccio sulla schiena o sul collo. Lasciatelo sciogliere.

• **Criosauna.** Una sessione di un paio di minuti costa circa 10 euro. Guarda in un centro specializzato.

Come eseguire il raffreddamento per le persone esperte?

- **Secchio sulla testa**. Riempire il secchio con acqua fredda. Vai fuori o sotto la doccia. Versare sulla testa. L'impatto è molto breve nel tempo, ma molto acuto nella forza.

- **Immersione completa**. Riempi la vasca con acqua fredda e immergi completamente il tuo corpo, tranne la testa, sotto l'acqua.

- **Doccia di contrasto 2 min**. Porta un orologio sotto l'acqua fredda per 240 secondi. Quindi è necessario alternare 120 secondi per il freddo e 60-120 secondi per il caldo. Finiamo sempre a freddo.

- **Solo una doccia fredda 5 min**. Non usiamo affatto l'acqua calda. Immediatamente entrare nell'acqua fredda e tenerla per 5 minuti.

- **Immergere il piede/la mano nella neve**. Riempire la bacinella di neve e metterci le mani per 2 minuti. Dopo questo, fare lo stesso per le gambe.

- **Spremere la neve**. Prendere una manciata di neve tra le mani e poi strofinarla sul corpo (braccia, spalle, petto, gambe, viso, ecc.).

●**Camicia bagnata**. Immergere la camicia in acqua ghiacciata e metterla su un corpo nudo. Qui si può progredire nell'impatto. 2-3 minuti sono un buon risultato per iniziare. In futuro, si può aumentare.

●**Camminare per strada**. Vai a fare una passeggiata/corsa in abbigliamento leggero (pantaloncini, maglietta) a una temperatura inferiore a 10 C. L'obiettivo è 5-10 minuti.

●**Camminare senza scarpe**. Camminare a piedi nudi a temperature inferiori a 10 C.

●**Criosauna**. Chiedere di aumentare l'impatto del freddo.

Cosa succede se espongo il corpo subito nel massimo freddo?

Lo stress può essere grande e lo stress può essere lungo. Tuttavia, allo stesso tempo (grande e lungo stress) può essere pericoloso perché il tuo corpo non è esattamente adattato a simili effetti. La temperatura molto fredda è un grande stress (perché è molto fredda). Immergersi in questo stress per un paio di minuti senza allenamento è una cattiva idea. Si può facilmente prendere un raffreddore e ammalarsi. Tuttavia, puoi immergerti in uno stress simile per un paio di secondi. Questa è una strategia valida.

Qual la miglior sauna?

Dipende dai tuoi obiettivi. Se volete influenzare tutto il vostro corpo in generale, vale la pena prestare attenzione alla SAUNA INFRAROSSI. Il fatto è che le saune tradizionali/bagno turco non riscaldano in modo uniforme il nostro corpo. Prima di tutto, la pelle e i muscoli sono riscaldati. Gli organi interni vengono riscaldati per ultimi. E se la temperatura è molto alta, allora non c'è tempo per riscaldarsi perché bisogna interrompere la procedura.

Qual è il tempo sufficiente per la sauna?

Ci sono dati che dicono che, se si fa il bagno turco o la sauna ogni giorno, si ottengono più benefici che se lo si fa una volta alla settimana. Capisco perfettamente che la pratica è abbastanza difficile da attuare. L'approccio più sensato sarebbe quello di usare la sauna IR tre volte alla settimana. Questa opzione è ideale per te se vai in un fitness club/palestra dove c'è una sauna a infrarossi.

In ogni caso, potrete comprare una piccola sauna acquistabile a un centinaio di euro. La durata dev'essere di 15 minuti circa.

Capitolo 3

BIOHAKING STILE DI VITA

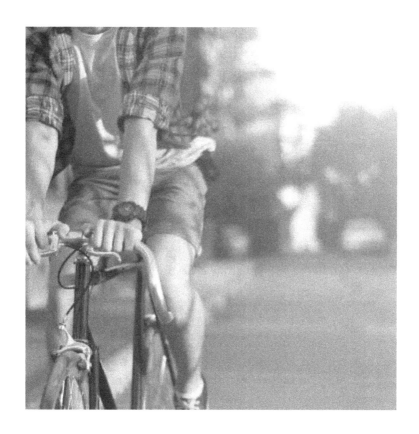

Recupero della Colonna Cervicale

La colonna cervicale è difficile da migliorare senza ripristinare tutta la colonna. Lo yoga fa bene. Affinché gli esercizi non siano eseguiti invano, dobbiamo aiutare il nostro corpo a riparare le vertebre del collo danneggiate. È necessario regolare il flusso di nutrienti e ormoni adeguati nel sangue. Una buona alimentazione e il digiuno periodico ci aiuteranno in questo (descritti in seguito). In questo capitolo, oltre agli esercizi di rafforzamento generale e al ripristino della posizione normale delle vertebre, troverete anche diverse tecniche che vi aiuteranno in casi di emergenza durante un attacco di panico. Voglio anche far notare che, il processo di recupero completo, può richiedere da sei mesi a due anni, ma già dalla prima settimana sentirete un significativo sollievo, e gli attacchi di panico si indeboliranno o spariranno completamente.

Esercizi che dovresti fare ogni mattina.

Ogni mattina, prima di mangiare, si dovrebbero fare 2 esercizi molto semplici.

1)   Gira la testa a sinistra e a destra per 250 cicli.

2)   Secondo. Inclinazione della testa avanti e indietro per 250 cicli.

Questi esercizi sono molto semplici tecnicamente, ma all'inizio possono essere complicati quantitativamente. Cercate di non farvi male, se durante questo vi sentite storditi o siete stanchi, fate una breve pausa e continuate dopo l'esercizio. Le curve e i piegamenti devono essere eseguiti rapidamente e bruscamente (naturalmente, tenendo conto delle vostre capacità, del dolore e delle restrizioni di movimento), ma allo stesso tempo con attenzione e non attraverso il dolore. Se la capacità di ruotare il collo è limitata, allora fai giri e piegamenti fino alla metà del possibile. La cosa principale è lavorare sulla quantità. È consigliabile arrivare a fare tutte le 250 volte senza una pausa.

Questo esercizio permette di rafforzare i muscoli del collo, riscaldare e attirare più sangue alle nostre vertebre cervicali, mettere gradualmente a posto le nostre vertebre e ripristinare il loro corretto funzionamento. Dopo un paio di settimane, la mobilità del collo aumenterà, e dopo circa un mese, gli scricchiolii cominceranno a scomparire.

Esercizi che dovresti fare due volte a settimana.

Preferibilmente farle dopo lo yoga o dopo aver raddrizzato la colonna vertebrale.

1) Sedersi in una posizione comoda, appoggiare le mani sui fianchi e cercare di allungare la colonna vertebrale. Si deve allungare per circa 30 secondi, poi, senza cambiare la posizione, si deve raddrizzare il collo, usando i muscoli del trapezio. Poi inclimiamo la testa verso il basso, e cominciamo poi a sollevarla lentamente e a gettarla indietro, appoggiando gradualmente le nostre vertebre contro i muscoli del trapezio tesi, e quindi impostando e allungando le vertebre cervicali.

2) Sedersi in una posizione comoda con la schiena dritta. Girare la testa a destra e tenerla in questa posizione per un minuto e mezzo. Ripeti l'esercizio girando la testa a sinistra. Si può sentire un leggero intorpidimento in una delle mani in questo momento. Questo indica una vertebra spostata e lo spostamento dei nervi. Se l'intorpidimento è tollerato e non si esprime chiaramente, allora non farci caso. Questo esercizio stabilizza le vertebre e rafforza i muscoli del collo.

3)   Successivamente, si può correggere leggermente il collo. Forse avete visto come un terapista manuale fa una procedura simile. Voi stessi potete fare questa procedura, ma non fatela spesso. Al massimo due volte alla settimana. In caso di emergenza con un attacco di panico, metti l'interno del palmo della mano destra sulla parte inferiore del mento sul lato sinistro, e con la mano sinistra afferri il lato destro della testa proprio sopra l'orecchio (o viceversa) con la punta delle dita e fai movimenti leggeri ma netti, come se volessi girare il collo. Si possono fare diversi movimenti di questo tipo per regolare la forza dello scatto.

Durante questa procedura, si può sentire un leggero scricchiolio. Più forte è lo scricchiolio, più problematico è il collo. Non abbiate paura di rompere il collo. Se fate tutto senza problemi e facilmente, allora il vostro collo e i vostri muscoli non si romperanno. Se questo esercizio ti provoca dolore, dovresti rimandarlo per un mese o due. Con il tempo, la crosta dovrebbe diventare sempre meno dura.

4)   Nella stessa postura seduta con la schiena piatta, inclinate la testa verso la spalla (tirate la testa di lato mentre guardate dritto davanti a voi). Allo stesso tempo dal lato opposto tirate la mano verso il pavimento. Con l'altra mano, si può afferrare la testa (con la punta delle dita sopra l'orecchio) e quindi allungare delicatamente il collo per non più di 30 secondi. Fate entrambi i modi.

Esercizi per l'auto-educazione delle vertebre

Raccomando di non fare questi esercizi inutilmente, ma di farli con molta attenzione. In nessun caso, non farli più di una volta al mese. Se li fai troppo spesso, puoi causare una destabilizzazione artificiale delle vertebre. Il complesso di esercizi sopra elencati, ti permette di allineare, rafforzare e stabilizzare gradualmente le vertebre e dovrebbe essere sufficiente per ripristinare la colonna cervicale. Ma in alcuni casi è necessaria una correzione più profonda del collo. Ancora una volta vi avverto che potete farlo non più di una volta al mese, a vostro rischio e pericolo, e dopo aver consultato il vostro medico prima. Dopo questo complesso, è necessario sdraiarsi per circa un'ora e durante il giorno cercare di non sforzare molto il collo.

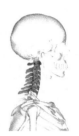

Step 1 - Riscaldare e modificare tutto il collo con un'espressione sulle vertebre C5-C7.

1)   Movimenti circolari con le spalle indietro (30-60 sec.);

2)   Movimenti circolari con le spalle in avanti (30-60 sec.);

3)   Scrollata di spalle su e giù (30-60 sec.);

4)   Movimenti circolari delle mani in avanti (30-40 sec.);

5)   Movimenti circolari delle braccia indietro (30-40 sec.);

6)   Oscillare le mani in verticale (una mano su e indietro, l'altra giù e indietro e viceversa) (30-40 sec.);

7)   Comprimere le braccia come una posa da boxe, poi sciogliere la schiena e le braccia piegate ai gomiti (20-30 volte);

8)   Mani all'altezza del petto, torsioni della schiena a sinistra e a destra insieme al collo e alla testa (20-30 volte);

9)   Strofinare i muscoli della cervicale con il palmo della mano, mentre ci si aiuta girando la testa (30-40 sec);

10)   Massaggio dei muscoli posteriori del collo con la punta delle dita (30 sec);

11)   Premiamo con i polpastrelli i muscoli suboccipitali e le vertebre, mentre con i palmi delle mani stabilizziamo il collo e facciamo movimenti di annuire con la testa inclinata all'indietro (20 sec);

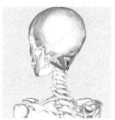

12)   Mettiamo il medio e l'indice sotto la nuca e facciamo movimenti di annuire con la testa inclinata all'indietro (20 sec);

13)   Fare un cenno a sinistra con la testa alla spalla per 3-4 secondi, poi girare la testa a destra alla spalla destra. Facciamo 5-7 volte, poi nell'altra direzione;

14)   Si inclina la testa verso la spalla (tirare la testa di lato mentre si guarda dritto). Con l'altra mano, afferrate la testa (con i polpastrelli sopra l'orecchio) e quindi allungate delicatamente il collo per non più di 30 secondi. Fate in entrambi i modi;

15)   Con il dito medio (se volete insieme all'indice) di una mano (o entrambe le mani se necessario) premiamo fortemente la fossetta suboccipitale proprio in mezzo. Poi fate movimenti di annuire con la testa all'indietro (20 sec);

16)   Tirare (trazione) il collo verso l'alto con le mani (30 sec).

Step 2 - Autocorrezione della colonna cervicale.

1)   Si fa un riscaldamento del collo dal complesso precedente (da 1 a 10);

2)   Si mettono i pollici tra gli zigomi (sotto le orecchie, dove la mascella si collega con il collo). Il resto delle dita messe sulla testa. Inspirando, tratteniamo il respiro e premiamo con i pollici per 10 secondi. Espirare. Così facciamo 2-4 cicli;

3)   Inclinare la testa indietro e di lato per 5 secondi, poi anche dall'altra parte;

4)   Una mano tiene il collo da dietro sotto l'orecchio, l'altra mano tira la parte superiore della testa nella direzione opposta con scatti leggeri. Fare così per 5-6 volte su entrambi i lati del collo;

5)   Ora, al contrario, la mano destra spinge il collo a destra, la mano sinistra spinge a sinistra. Fare per 5-6 volte, poi si cambia lato;

6)   Mettiamo il pollice sotto le orecchie, dove la mascella si unisce al collo. Premiamo e facciamo movimenti della testa avanti e indietro per 10-12 volte;

7)   Gettare fortemente indietro la testa, allungare il mento verso l'alto. In questa posizione, girare la testa assialmente a destra e a sinistra; raccomando anche vivamente la trazione (estensione) del collo nelle fasi iniziali del recupero.

È molto utile anche dormire senza un cuscino. Così, sdraiato sulla schiena, il collo è nella posizione anatomicamente corretta. E se ci si sdraia sul fianco, quando la testa pende verso il basso, automaticamente si allunga e si raddrizza il collo durante le 6-8 ore di sonno, il che porta all'inevitabile raddrizzamento graduale e al ripristino delle vertebre spostate. Dopo sei mesi di pratica di tale sonno, ho notato un effetto positivo, ovvero un sonno più profondo, il collo non si intorpidisce, la testa è chiara al mattino e lo stato è allegro. Inoltre, a causa di problemi al collo, ho avuto problemi di pressione alta e a volte, quando la testa non era posizionata correttamente durante il sonno, al mattino ho osservato un aumento della pressione e mi sono sentito sopraffatto.

Così, dopo aver praticato il sonno senza cuscino, questo problema è scomparso completamente. Forse questo metodo non è adatto a qualcuno e non porterà così tanti benefici, ma vi assicuro che vale la pena provare. E ancora una volta voglio avvertirvi che se qualche esercizio vi causa dolore, dovreste eseguirlo più delicatamente o metterlo da parte per un po'.

Hack Sonno

Il sonno è fondamentale. Durante il sonno si produce l'ormone GH (ormone anti-invecchiamento) che incrementa aumento massa muscolare, testosterone, stimola l'ormone dal fegato GF-1, non sfasa i ritmi circadiani, diminuisce il rischio di malattie, stimola una mente più lucida e tanto altro. Non dormire nell'orario giusto, con un sonno di qualità e il giusto quantitativo di ore ha conseguenze su tutto l'organismo e sfasa il ritmo circadiano. La produzione di melatonina va massimizzata per garantirsi piena salute e massima energia. La melatonina, oltre ad essere l'ormone del sonno, è anche un antiossidante e regola il ritmo circadiano.

Bisogna incentivarne la produzione e non assumerla come integratore. Questo perché la produzione naturale è quella migliore, in quanto l'organismo sa quanta crearne e quanto ne è necessaria nel corpo. Questo non può avvenire con quella artificiale.

Cos'è il ritmo circadiano?

Il ritmo circadiano è una sorta di orologio biologico, il cui periodo è di 24 ore.
Ogni giorno si ripetono periodicamente determinate condizioni nel

nostro corpo, come ad esempio il ritmo sonno-veglia. L'orologio circadiano è un complesso sistema interno regolato da molti fattori e basato su stimoli provenienti dall'esterno. Ad esempio il ritmo di sonno veglia è regolato in base alla luce e alla temperatura dell'ambiente. Il sistema che sta alla base della regolazione di questo ritmo è controllato da un gruppo di cellule situate in una regione dell'ipotalamo. Secondo studi di scienziati ogni giorno è suddiviso in cicli di 3 ore, durante i quali il nostro organismo è portato a fare certi esercizi o attività piuttosto che altre.

- Ore 6:00-8:59
  È il ciclo in cui il corpo gradualmente si rimette in moto. La produzione di melatonina cessa.

- Ore 9.00-11.59
  In questo ciclo il cortisolo raggiunge il suo picco e lo stato di concentrazione e attivazione dell'organismo è massimo. È il momento migliore per svolgere le incombenze più impegnative della giornata. Ovviamente qui è sconsigliato dormire.

- Ore 12.00-14:59
  In queste 3 ore l'attività digestiva determina sonnolenza. Cerca di non bere alcolici e concediti invece una passeggiata per digerire, o una breve siesta.

- Ore 15.00-17:59
  Sono le ore ideali per concentrarsi sull'attività fisica, perché la temperatura corporea aumenta naturalmente, e cuore e polmoni raggiungono il massimo della loro efficienza.

- Ore 18.00-20:59
  È l'orario adatto per la cena, ma senza eccedere.

- Ore 21.00-23:59
  In questo ciclo si inizia a produrre la melatonina, la temperatura corporea inizia a scendere, ed è giunto il

momento di infilarsi a letto. Evita di fare sport o di stare sullo smartphone.

- Ore 3.00-5:59
  È l'ultimo ciclo, durante il quale è consigliato dormire.

Come ottimizzare la produzione di melatonina?

Durante il giorno dobbiamo "bloccare" la produzione di melatonina. Quindi bisogna alzarci ad un orario decente, stare il più possibile alla luce ed evitare luoghi bui, stare al sole nei momenti "chiave" della giornata (orari dalle 07-09 e dalle 12 / 18).

Di sera dobbiamo incentivare la produzione di melatonina. Quindi evitare il più possibile l'illuminazione (evitare luce blu, ma va bene la luce rossa). Di notte, per favorire anche in questo momento la produzione di melatonina, dormire completamente al buio e lontano dai disturbi (basta una fonte di luce per alterare la produzione. Varia in base all'intensità della luce). Non basta mettersi maschere di notte perché anche la pelle ne risente.

Perché il sonno non deve essere "disturbato"?

Ecco cosa implica:

- Alterazione del ritmo circadiano.
- Aumento cortisolo.
- Diminuzione del testosterone.
- Diminuzione di melatonina.
- Diminuzione ormone della crescita.
- Disfunzione del sistema linfatico.
- Perdita memoria, concentrazione e capacità cognitive.
- Aumento resistenza all'insulina.

- Aumento rischio di contrarre cancro.
- Bassa energia.
- Mancato respiro.
- Altro...

Cosa fare per avere un sonno buono?

- Evita docce fredde nelle ore serali in quanto eccitante (fare bagno caldo con sali di magnesio).
- Dalle 19 in poi, appena cala il sole, utilizza solo illuminazione rossa, fuoco, candele.
- Non ascoltare musica movimentata e rilassati bene.
- Stop dispositivi elettronici (leggi un libro).
- Spegni il wi-fi in casa.
- Non allenarti dopo le 17, se fai sport lattacidi anticipa ulteriormente.
- Non cenare tardi (non più tardi delle 19).
- Assicurati di non essere carente di vitamina D, retinolo e omega 3.
- Dormire al buio.
- La stanza non deve essere nè troppo calda né troppo fredda (18 – 22 °C).
- Aumenta il riscaldamento d'inverno se necessario e usa ventilatore d'estate.
- Evita rumori molesti.
- Utilizza uno ionizzatore per l'aria da installare nella stanza per arricchirla di elettroni e privarla di impurità (gli elettroni creano serotonina che la sera si converte in melatonina).
- Utilizza un materasso e cuscino appropriati.
- Metti il telefono in modalità "aerea" oppure allontanalo da te circa 1,5 - 2 metri.
- Vai a dormire prima delle 23. Consigliato di mettersi a letto alle 21.30, leggere un libro e spegnere le luci rosse quando arriva il sonno.

- Stare a distanza con il letto almeno 30 - 40 cm da prese elettriche (in quanto creano campi elettromagnetici).
- Meditare prima di dormire.
- Ascoltare toni binaurali.
- Evitare caffè e sostanze eccitanti nella seconda parte della giornata.

L'ideale sarebbe svegliarsi la mattina senza sveglia, avendo riposato 8-9 ore a notte.

Capitolo 4

SISTEMA NERVOSO CENTRALE E BIOHACKING

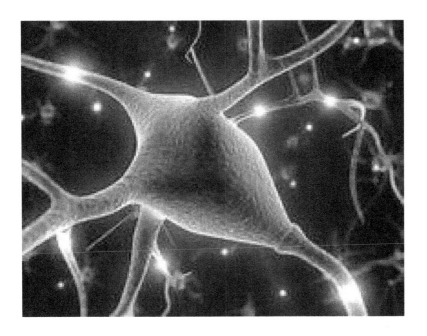

Forse non è possibile dimostrarlo scientificamente, ma il Sistema Nervoso Centrale è vita. Puoi sentirlo, ma devi essere attento.

Sentire il tuo SNC

Spesso, anzi quasi sempre, sono i nostri organi sensoriali, come gli occhi, le orecchie, la pelle, ecc. che ci danno il senso se il nostro sistema nervoso funziona correttamente o no. Quando funziona correttamente in modo ottimale, non sentiamo alcuna differenza o anomalia. Solo quando c'è un malfunzionamento da qualche parte, riceviamo avvisi sotto forma di sintomi che indicano che si è verificato un errore. Come un disco che si è bloccato! Se siete all'erta, i sintomi generalmente iniziano come vaghe sensazioni di intorpidimento o formicolio, fino a quando non inizia a peggiorare, e il vero problema inizia. Anche se ci possono essere altri sintomi iniziali, in generale sono intorpidimento e formicolio. Sono i più visibili e riportati.

L'intorpidimento implica nessuna sensazione, mentre il formicolio implica la sensazione di punture di spillo in quella zona. Sia l'intorpidimento che il formicolio, indicano una bandiera rossa nel tuo SNC.

Stress - non è nel tuo cervello, è nel tuo sistema nervoso

Il nostro sistema nervoso reagisce allo stress attraverso il sistema nervoso *parasimpatico* e quello *simpatico*. Quando ci si trova sotto emozioni negative, come la rabbia o la paura, il braccio simpatico del nostro SNC reagisce, preparando il corpo ad affrontare il pericolo percepito. In quel caso, il nostro sistema nervoso simpatico fornisce anche al corpo una sferzata di energia in modo che possa rispondere con una reazione di 'lotta o fuga' alle minacce percepite.

Gli ormoni dello stress, come il cortisolo e l'adrenalina, vengono rilasciati dalla ghiandola surrenale. Questi ormoni causano un effetto immediato sugli organi vitali del nostro corpo e li preparano ad eseguire la decisione presa, cioè lotta o fuga. Alcuni dei più comuni sono: il cuore comincia a battere più velocemente, la respirazione aumenta, il processo digestivo cambia, ecc. Una volta che la situazione stressante è finita, il corpo comincia a tornare alla condizione pre-emergenza con tutti gli organi vitali che riprendono le loro funzioni normali.

Lo *stress cronico* è spesso un'abitudine mentale debilitante, quando una persona cade nella routine di percepire tutto e qualsiasi cosa accada nella sua vita con un quadro negativo. È lo stress interminabile che comincia a prendere di mira il SNC. Senza speranza, l'individuo alla fine rinuncia a cercare soluzioni valide, e col passare del tempo si rassegna a vivere a quel livello di stress. Alcuni stress cronici possono derivare da esperienze traumatiche della prima infanzia che vengono interiorizzate e rimangono incastrate nella nostra psiche per far rivivere il ricordo di un passato doloroso nella vita presente. Il ricordo di tale stress cronico spesso rimane per un lungo periodo di tempo. Lo stress cronico può gradualmente logorare le risorse della mente e del corpo. Infatti, la pressione di tale stress è stata medicalmente collegata a malattie cardiache, pressione alta, colesterolo alto e depressione. Le ricerche fisiologiche dimostrano che la memoria della risposta allo stress vive incorporata nel nostro sistema nervoso, poiché una delle responsabilità funzionali chiave del SNC è quella di immagazzinare e trasportare fedelmente le emozioni.

Malattie Psicosomatiche e il SNC

Le malattie psicosomatiche e le malattie del SNC, come l'ulcera allo stomaco, l'artrite, l'infiammazione e le parti del corpo gonfie, non hanno un punto di partenza concreto, ma possono infiammarsi in condizioni di stress continuo o prolungato. A mio parere, esistono due tipi principali di stress. Uno che è visibile o che possiamo sentire attraverso i nostri sensi - occhi, orecchie, pelle, ecc.-. Questi sono chiaramente percepibili. L'altro è lo stress invisibile, come le radiazioni elettromagnetiche, i cui effetti negativi non si percepiscono immediatamente con nessuno dei nostri organi sensoriali. Nel momento in cui il nostro corpo è sotto stress, il SNC crea un drenaggio temporaneo di energia dalle riserve del corpo per affrontare le situazioni di stress. L'unico obiettivo del nostro SNC è quello di proteggere e guarire il corpo da qualsiasi tipo di stress.

Quando siamo sotto uno o entrambi i tipi di stress, dopo un certo tempo, il nostro SNC cerca di proteggere il corpo da tutti i pericoli percepiti e per questo non richiede alcuna istruzione dal nostro cervello o dal midollo spinale. Infatti, il SNC ha un'intelligenza incorporata per iniziare la guarigione. Così, all'interno del nostro corpo, il SNC inizia il suo lavoro di guarigione da solo. Ma nei casi in cui il fattore di stress rimane presente nella nostra vita per un periodo di tempo relativamente lungo, il potere del SNC di guarire e riparare si esaurisce e perde la sua potenza. Questi sono i momenti in cui si verificano le malattie psicosomatiche e certe malattie dello stile di vita come l'artrite, l'ulcera allo stomaco, ecc.

Queste malattie sono esempi classici in cui il SNC sta ancora lavorando per guarire il corpo, ma è a corto di energia per farlo. La fibromialgia è il secondo disturbo reumatico più comune dopo l'osteoartrite, ed è ormai considerato un disturbo del SNC. In questo caso, la persona che ne soffre può sentire un dolore amplificato che picchia nel suo corpo.

Emozioni e SNC

È mia forte convinzione che le emozioni rimangano confinate nel SNC. Quando una persona non è in grado di elaborare e rilasciare le emozioni negative, il risultato è un trauma. Se le emozioni rimangono irrisolte nel SNC, l'intensità di quell'evento traumatico comincerebbe a creare blocchi nei percorsi energetici e interferire con il normale funzionamento di esso.

Durante questi momenti traumatici, il SNC cerca prima di tutto di guarire sé stesso. Questo è il momento in cui osserviamo le malattie autoimmuni come l'artrite e/o le parti del corpo gonfie, che fanno la loro prima comparsa. La stessa logica si applica ad altre parti del corpo. Per esempio, secondo la medicina tradizionale cinese la rabbia è collegata al fegato. Quando ci sono problemi di rabbia repressa o irrisolta, il sistema nervoso del fegato cercherà innanzitutto di guarire sé stesso, ma quando la situazione va oltre il suo controllo, la sua capacità e il suo potere di guarire falliscono, e il risultato potrebbe essere la cirrosi epatica e l'insufficienza epatica.

Come il SNC inizia a bloccarsi e le persone invecchiano nel tempo

Essenzialmente, il ruolo del SNC è quello di far circolare liberamente l'energia in tutto il corpo. Tuttavia, nel corso del tempo, possono svilupparsi blocchi nel percorso di questo libero flusso di energia a causa di traumi o stress. La risposta intuitiva del SNC è di guarire sé stesso inviando energia alla parte afflitta.

A seconda della forte energia del SNC della persona, il suo recupero dalla malattia può essere completo o parziale. Se la guarigione è completa, la parte malata guarisce completamente e l'energia ricomincia a muoversi liberamente, senza impedimenti. Generalmente troviamo questo tratto molto forte nei bambini, ed è per questo che guariscono più velocemente e completamente da qualsiasi malattia. Mentre il SNC sta ancora lavorando, il cervello e il midollo spinale possono non avere idea di cosa stia succedendo, poiché l'energia in un corpo umano è fissa e limitata e deve fluire anche in altre parti vitali del corpo. In questo modo, una o più parti del corpo o una parte del SNC si "bloccano" e diventano rigide. In sostanza, le persone invecchiano non per le leggi della natura, ma perché con il tempo, il loro SNC e le parti del corpo iniziano a congelarsi attraverso il processo spiegato sopra.

Questo fenomeno continua da una parte del corpo all'altra; da un'area del SNC all'altra, e alla fine perdiamo tutta l'energia vitale assegnataci al momento della nascita, e cominciamo ad invecchiare, fino a perdere tutta l'energia e morire. La ragione per cui ho scritto questo libro è di spiegarvi come potete 'hackerare' la biologia del vostro corpo con l'aiuto del biohacking e del SNC e mantenere sempre una salute ottimale e raggiungere la longevità. Quando si tratta di una questione emotiva negativa che generalmente non "lasciamo andare", cominciamo a sperimentare una tale tensione intorno e dentro le zone dell'intestino crasso e dell'intestino tenue. Questa è una ragione abbastanza grande per cui dovremmo mantenere il nostro intestino pulito e forte. La cosa peggiore che succede quando hai ricordi traumatici alloggiati nel SNC è che quest'ultimo comincia a esaurire le risorse energetiche del tuo corpo, minuto per minuto senza che tu nemmeno lo sappia.

Reagisce a quel trauma residuo costantemente. Questo è il motivo per cui raccomando che ogni ricordo traumatico deve essere rilasciato dal tuo corpo per salvare e conservare la tua energia vitale.

Dolore e SNC

Il SNC informa il cervello sul dolore. In realtà, è il SNC che sente e trasporta il dolore. Se il SNC è pienamente attivo, allora è del tutto possibile per noi non provare alcun dolore. Una vita senza dolore è il simbolo di un SNC pienamente funzionante e senza blocchi.

Biohacking e SNC

Hai mai sentito il detto: *"Tu sei quello che mangi"?*

Qualunque cosa metti nel tuo corpo (il cibo, i pensieri o i movimenti fisici), influenzano il tuo modo di comportarti. Tuttavia, questa biologia del tuo corpo è ancora modificabile se sei pronto a fare alcuni cambiamenti al tuo stile di vita. Ed è qui che entra in gioco il biohacking. Esso è un modo di trasformare il tuo corpo con il chiaro obiettivo di aumentare i tuoi livelli di energia, migliorare la tua produttività e sentirti la migliore versione di te stesso. Non c'è bisogno di cercare scienziati che facciano esperimenti folli sul tuo corpo. Tutto quello che devi fare è esplorare i vari hack condivisi, e scoprire cosa funziona meglio per te.

Ma lasciatemi prima confessare come mi sono imbattuto nella parola biohacking. È stato menzionato per la prima volta nel 1988 in un articolo pubblicato sul Washington Post. Più tardi il termine fu raffinato e introdotto come un processo di "manipolazione del codice genetico di un organismo vivente". Gli esperti moderni, come Dave Asprey e Ben Greenfield, considerano il biohacking un'arte più che una scienza. Secondo Dave Asprey, il biohacking è un approccio sistemico che si può usare per hackerare la propria biologia. In primo luogo siamo d'accordo che il tuo corpo è un sistema che riceve input definiti, come il cibo e l'esercizio fisico, e output, come l'energia e l'umore. Modificando o mettendo a punto gli input che entrano nel vostro sistema, potete causare cambiamenti istantanei e misurabili nei vostri output.

Devi provare per scoprire cosa succede; e poi puoi iniziare a prendere le tue decisioni.

Tipi di Biohacking

Ci sono tre categorie nel Biohacking: La nutrigenomica, la biologia fai-da-te, e il grinder biohacking.

La nutrigenomica si riferisce allo studio della manipolazione dell'attività del tuo corpo attraverso la nutrizione. Coinvolge anche la manipolazione del sonno, l'hacking dell'attenzione, l'esercizio, la gestione dello stress e l'adattamento ai trigger ambientali, come il suono e la luce. La nutrigenomica crede nel concetto che la funzione del corpo e la nutrigenomica possono essere alterate attraverso il cibo, l'attività e altri stimoli. Si tratta di scoprire questi cambiamenti e usarli per vivere meglio. Vedremo in seguito, nel dettaglio, cosa mangiare o meno.

La biologia fai-da-te si concentra sullo studio e la sperimentazione della scienza del biohacking che non è provata. Questi biohacker, che di solito sono ricercatori scientifici ed educatori formali, conducono esperimenti biologici non convenzionali per studiare le scienze della vita e insegnano ai profani come condurre questi esperimenti. Per quanto affascinanti possano sembrare i loro sforzi, sono spesso criticati dal resto del mondo, poiché non c'è una supervisione ufficiale.

Il grinder biohacking è una parte della biologia fai-da-te, che si concentra sulla manipolazione chimica del corpo e sugli impianti tecnologici. I grinder sono spesso coinvolti nella modifica del corpo e nel miglioramento del suo hardware, spingendo la tecnologia e la potenza del corpo umano oltre i limiti. L'approccio non è raccomandato poiché queste tecniche sembrano molto rischiose. È attraverso il vostro sistema nervoso che sperimentate la vostra vita. Il vostro sistema nervoso centrale è quello che coordina e controlla ogni pensiero, ogni respiro, ogni battito cardiaco, ogni movimento e ogni vostro ricordo. Se hai bisogno di biohackerare il tuo sistema, devi iniziare biohackerando il tuo sistema nervoso centrale. Questo è il nucleo di questo libro.

Hacking del tuo SNC

Hacking del tuo SNC consiste nel ripulirlo e attivarlo. L'attenzione deve essere focalizzata sulla pulizia del SNC, poiché la guarigione avverrà automaticamente. Il SNC è abbastanza potente da resettare sé stesso alla sua condizione originale, senza alcun aiuto esterno, purché abbia sufficiente energia. Le seguenti tecniche possono essere usate a questo scopo. E se per caso il vostro SNC è chiaro, allora queste tecniche vi aiuteranno ad aumentare i vostri poteri di esso

Respirazione a narici alternate

Questo è uno dei migliori e più semplici metodi per liberare il SNC. Questa è una tecnica che purifica le tue narici e permette all'energia di muoversi liberamente in tutto il corpo. Storicamente la respirazione a narici alternate era considerata un modo per armonizzare i due emisferi del cervello umano. Così facendo, puoi portare un equilibrio nel tuo benessere fisico, mentale ed emotivo. Ecco alcuni benefici della pratica di questa tecnica.

- Attiva il sistema nervoso parasimpatico
- Abbassa la pressione sanguigna.
- Migliora le tue funzioni respiratorie e aumenta la tua resistenza.
- Migliora l'attenzione e la coordinazione motoria.
- Migliora salute del cuore, dei polmoni e della testa.

Respirazione del grembo

La respirazione del grembo è una tecnica di respirazione inversa in cui si restringe la pancia mentre si inspira e la si espande mentre si espira. Ti riporta nel tuo centro primordiale, che è il tuo grembo (la tua coscienza femminile, i tuoi istinti, i tuoi sentimenti, e la tua creatura erotica del corpo). La tecnica ti intreccia di nuovo in una rete di coscienza che è filata dal grembo del creatore. Il processo si chiama "Risveglio del Grembo" che è un percorso di attaccamento e riconnessione radicale. Quando sei connesso al grembo ti senti assolutamente rilassato, infinitamente creativo e potente, radioso, energizzato, sostenuto dalla terra/universo, e connesso alla tua saggezza e piacere interiore.

Iniziate a sviluppare e rafforzare la fede o la fiducia dentro di voi.

Esercizio Tibetano

Il Rito Tibetano è un esercizio restrittivo che deve essere praticato solo se un soggetto sta avendo un eccessivo impulso sessuale. Il Rito Tibetano incanala l'energia sessuale o riproduttiva in eccesso verso i chakra superiori, specialmente il chakra della fronte, che regola le capacità psichiche e il risveglio spirituale. Il Rito Tibetano è un esercizio facile da eseguire, tenendo conto della prospettiva fisica. Tuttavia, poiché implica un prolungato trattenimento del respiro, potrebbe essere necessaria una certa pratica per perfezionare questa tecnica. Bisogna fare attenzione a non ripetere questo esercizio per più di tre volte al giorno.

Anche ogni ciclo del Rito Tibetano deve essere seguito da cicli ripetuti di respirazione profonda per ottenere risultati migliori.

Reiki

Il Reiki è una delle tecniche molto importanti che possono essere praticate per eliminare i blocchi nel SNC e attivarlo per fornire ulteriore energia di guarigione al corpo. Rei in giapponese significa "la Saggezza di Dio o il Potere Superiore", e Ki significa "l'energia della forza vitale". Il Reiki è il processo di guidare spiritualmente l'energia della forza vitale per ristabilire l'equilibrio e la vitalità nel corpo. Il Reiki aiuta ad alleviare il corpo dagli effetti fisici ed emotivi dello stress aprendo meridiani bloccati e liberando il flusso di energia.

Chiunque può attingere a questa forza vitale e migliorare la propria qualità di vita imparando il Reiki.

Forza Kundalini

La forza Kundalini è l'energia che è dormiente nel Muladhara. Se attivata e canalizzata correttamente, può eliminare tutti i blocchi nel SNC e fornire al corpo energia extra. L'esercizio di attivazione del potere Kundalini dovrebbe essere fatto solo sotto la guida di un insegnante o di un maestro professionista. Altrimenti potrebbe causare gravi danni.

Si dice che l'energia cosmica divina dorma alla base della spina dorsale in una forma arrotolata. Può essere sentita come una calda energia magnetica che sale dalla base della spina dorsale verso l'alto. Lungo il percorso di questa energia ci sono i sette chakra principali. Ognuno di questi centri si attiva e prende vita quando questa energia li attraversa. Quando la kundalini diventa più forte, puoi iniziare a sentire sensazioni simili a quelle di un serpente nella parte posteriore della spina dorsale. La Kundalini, quando viene attivata, ha il potere di curare mal di testa, insonnia, ansia e depressione, liberando il soggetto da disturbi mentali, problemi psichici e stress.

Portando i poteri psichici, la Kundalini stabilizza la mente, equilibra le emozioni e allevia il dolore e la sofferenza. Il risveglio della Kundalini è lo strumento definitivo per l'auto-miglioramento, che dà luogo a cambiamenti positivi a lungo termine. Tuttavia, una volta risvegliata non può essere trattenuta. Perciò è importante ottenere la guida di un insegnante illuminato.

Creare la realtà attraverso i pensieri

Ogni momento della giornata, il SNC continua a reagire fisicamente ai pensieri che attraversano la nostra mente. Secondo l'epigenetica, chi sei è il prodotto delle cose che ti succedono nella tua vita. Sono queste cose che cambiano il modo in cui operano i tuoi geni. I duri ricordi e lo stress non liberato, e le emozioni associate ai traumi che avete affrontato, tendono a trovarsi in profondità nel vostro SNC. Cambiando i vostri pensieri e le vostre percezioni, potete influenzare e modificare la vostra lettura genetica, nel modo che volete. Il modo per farlo è quello di hackerare il tuo SNC.

Hai mai sentito le parole: "*Se vuoi diventare il Padrone del tuo Destino, dovrai imparare a controllare la natura dei tuoi pensieri*"? È la vostra mente che forma, o definisce la materia. Dovrai usare i tuoi pensieri per incontrare la migliore versione di te.

Meditazione avanzata

La meditazione avanzata è la più potente di tutte. La meditazione è il modo migliore per permettere all'energia della forza vitale di fluire liberamente in tutto il corpo. Ha il potere di eliminare tutti i blocchi in tutti i luoghi, sia nel corpo fisico che in quello astrale. Migliaia di studi di ricerca scientifica hanno sostenuto gli illimitati benefici fisici, mentali e psicologici della meditazione.

Osservare il tuo corpo dall'esterno

Questo è uno dei modi migliori per controllare il tuo sistema nervoso centrale.

-    Siediti o sdraiati in una posizione comoda.
-    Chiudi gli occhi e inizia a fare alcuni respiri profondi.

- Immagina di guardare il tuo corpo da davanti o da qualsiasi angolo della stanza.

Non stai facendo altro che guardarti dall'esterno del tuo corpo. È uno dei modi migliori per eliminare i blocchi lungo il percorso dell'energia e attivare il potere del tuo corpo.

Se trovi difficile praticare questa tecnica, ce n'è un'altra che puoi provare appena prima di andare a letto.

- Sdraiati sul tuo letto in una posizione comoda.
- Chiudi gli occhi e fai qualche respiro profondo.
- Ora ricorda semplicemente tutto quello che è successo da quando ti sei svegliato la mattina fino a quando sei andato a letto.

Devi solo guardare gli eventi come se stessi guardando un film. Non dovete reagire a nulla. Questo è un metodo efficace per liberarsi di tutti i vostri blocchi emotivi negativi del giorno e pulire il vostro sistema nervoso centrale.

Respirare dal chakra dell'ombelico

Questo è il primo chakra che viene influenzato dalle tue emozioni negative e dalle tue reazioni di lotta o fuga. Il secondo cervello è nell'intestino, si riferisce a questo chakra. Puoi seguire questi passi per praticare la tecnica della respirazione dal chakra dell'ombelico.

- Sdraiati comodamente su un tappetino.
- Chiudi gli occhi e fai un paio di respiri profondi.
- Ora metti il palmo sinistro sopra l'ombelico e il palmo destro sopra il palmo sinistro.
- Concentrati sul tuo respiro per circa 10 minuti

Questo dovrebbe aiutarti a liberare questo chakra e quindi il tuo SNC. Oltre a migliorare la tua digestione, questa tecnica può anche aumentare la tua autostima e motivarti a condurre una vita soddisfacente. Fidati del tuo istinto e lavora su di esso per sviluppare e aprire il tuo chakra dell'ombelico. Comprendi la fonte del tuo disagio e scopri come puoi guarirlo naturalmente.

Silenzio profondo

Il silenzio profondo ha un effetto ringiovanente sul tuo SNC. È come il pulsante di 'reset' che porta il SNC alla sua condizione originale, eliminando tutti i blocchi. Per un effetto migliore, è necessario osservare il "silenzio profondo" per almeno 30 minuti. Questo è pieno di beatitudine. Per ascoltare questa musica silenziosa, dovrai abbandonare tutti i tuoi pensieri e diventare un osservatore della tua mente. Non c'è bisogno di ripeterla. Sii semplicemente silenzioso e ascoltalo affiorare da dentro di te. Quando la tua mente comincia a diventare calma e silenziosa, dovresti diventare consapevole di qualcosa come un sussurro. Ha una qualità totalmente diversa quando sorge da solo. Nel momento in cui raggiungete uno stato in cui potete sentire questo suono, significa che siete entrati nel profondo dei segreti dell'esistenza. Diventi assolutamente sottile. È questo momento di serenità che è la vera fragranza della meditazione. Nasce dal vuoto assoluto dove non ci sono pensieri e desideri. È una tecnica di disintossicazione che pulisce tutte le tossine che avete accumulato nel vostro corpo.

Yoga Nidra

Lo Yoga Nidra è un modo molto efficace per eliminare i blocchi dal SNC, specialmente quelli che sono legati alle tue memorie emotive e traumatiche. Lo Yoga Nidra ci aiuta ad accedere lo stato parasimpatico dove avviene la guarigione. Aumentando la consapevolezza del nostro corpo, ci aiuta a riposare, a de-stressarci e a ripristinare, aiutandoci infine a capire la nostra vera vocazione. Yoga Nidra è conosciuto come un metodo di rilassamento senza sforzo che può essere praticato da chiunque, ovunque. Consiste nel portare la vostra attenzione su diverse parti del vostro corpo e rilassarle. Si è assolutamente coscienti e consapevoli per tutto il tempo.

Sonno notturno

Questa è una tecnica che puoi praticare quando vai a letto la sera. Consiste nel rilassare il corpo e la mente, concentrandosi sul punto centrale tra le due sopracciglia. A differenza dello Yoga Nidra, questo non comporta alcuna istruzione o il rilascio forzato dello stress da qualsiasi parte del corpo. È un metodo altamente efficace che si concentra solo sulla concentrazione e sul sonno. La pratica regolare della tecnica del sonno notturno può fermare lo stress e aiutarvi a controllare il suo flusso in tutto il corpo. Inoltre libera e attiva il SNC.

Hacking dell'emozioni

Questa tecnica si concentra sullo svuotamento delle memorie profonde e sul rilascio delle emozioni ad esse associate.

- Siediti o sdraiati in una posizione comoda.
- Chiudi delicatamente gli occhi e fai qualche respiro profondo.
- Ora ricorda l'incidente traumatico che ti ha turbato di più e riproducilo nella tua mente senza giudicare o reagire.
- Guarda l'incidente come un estraneo e lascia andare le tue emozioni.

Sono i nostri ricordi che ci definiscono e alimentano le nostre più grandi ambizioni. Si trovano nella profondità delle nostre paure più oscure e sono quelli che permettono alla nostra mente di viaggiare dal presente al passato. Nascondere o sopprimere i tuoi ricordi traumatici potrebbe proteggerti dal dolore emotivo di ricordare l'evento. Tuttavia, a lungo andare, può portare a problemi psicologici debilitanti come la depressione, l'ansia e i disturbi dissociativi, come il disturbo post traumatico da stress.

Usare Suggerimenti Positivi e Creativi / Frequenze Sonore

Quando diamo suggerimenti positivi e creativi a noi stessi, essi raggiungeranno prima la nostra mente cosciente attraverso i nostri 5 sensi. Una volta che le suggestioni sono ricevute, la mente cosciente agisce su di esse. Decide poi cosa viene trasmesso alla mente subconscia agendo come un filtro. Usando il potere dei nostri pensieri e suggerimenti positivi, possiamo controllare completamente ciò che raggiunge la nostra mente subconscia e ciò che non lo fa. Rinforzare la vostra mente con affermazioni positive può aiutare a trasformare tutto il vostro mondo nel modo in cui volete che sia. Allo stesso modo puoi anche usare varie frequenze sonore per aiutare a eliminare i blocchi nel tuo SNC e attivare lo stesso. Gli studi hanno dimostrato che un maggior senso di equilibrio può essere raggiunto esponendosi a frequenze curative come la 528 Hz "Love Frequency" e la frequenza di 432 Hertz.

Ci sono molti che praticano la meditazione sonora per un rilassamento più rapido e profondo. Tutto quello che devi fare è usare la tua mente per stringere quella parte del tuo corpo e poi rilasciarla dopo 5 secondi. Sentite il flusso di energia e mandate il vostro respiro a quella parte del corpo. Una volta fatto, aspettate per 10 secondi e poi ripetete la tecnica. Potete ripetere questa tecnica per un massimo di 5 volte inizialmente. Questo eliminerà il blocco nel flusso di energia e aiuterà ad attivare il vostro SNC.

L'hacking del vostro sistema nervoso centrale è un modo molto efficace per guarire il vostro corpo e la vostra mente e raggiungere l'illuminazione spirituale. Anche se ci possono essere vari trattamenti per lo stesso, il modo migliore per farlo è proprio dentro di voi, nella vostra mente. Trova il modo migliore per rilassare il tuo corpo, riconosci i punti di stress dove l'energia può essere bloccata, rilascia lo stress attraverso i tuoi pensieri e senti il libero flusso di energia in tutto il corpo. Niente può essere paragonato alla beatitudine che sentirai una volta che il tuo SNC sarà chiaro e attivato.

Hacking toni binaurali

È ottimo da abbinare alla meditazione. I toni binaurali sono battimenti che vengono percepiti dal cervello quando due suoni con frequenza inferiore ai 1500 Hz e con differenza inferiore ai 30 Hz vengono ascoltati separatamente attraverso gli auricolari. Quindi ascoltiamo nell'auricolare di sinistra una frequenza di 1000 Hz, mentre nell'auricolare di destra ascoltiamo una frequenza di 1000 Hz meno 1-30 Hz (quindi 970-999 Hz).

Cosa succede? Noi non ci accorgiamo della differenza di suono tra le due orecchie (in quanto poca differenza), ma il cervello l'avverte la differenza e praticamente va a creare una terza frequenza che è la differenza tra le 2. Quindi il cervello creerà una nuova frequenza di 30 Hz. Questo fenomeno è stato identificato nel 1839 da Heinrich Wilhelm Dove.

A cosa serve? Servono per incanalare onde cerebrali specifiche. I neuroni comunicano mediante impulsi elettrici. I suoni binaurali sono delle particolari frequenze musicali che possono influenzare il nostro cervello portandolo in uno stato di apertura e coscienza tale da favorire la concentrazione, il rilassamento e l'apprendimento.

Onde elettromagnetiche cerebrali

Tutti gli stadi della nostra coscienza sono dovuti all'incessante attività elettrochimica del cervello, che si manifesta attraverso "onde elettromagnetiche", ovvero le onde cerebrali (misurano in Hz). La frequenza di tali onde varia a seconda del tipo di attività in cui il cervello è impegnato. L'attività cerebrale viene registrata attraverso l'elettro-encefalo-gamma (EEG) sotto-forma di onde misurate in Hz. Per tutto il giorno il nostro cervello mantiene attivi i 5 tipi di onde cerebrali. A seconda di quello che facciamo in ogni momento, ci saranno alcune onde che mostrano una maggiore attività in alcune aree del cervello e altre che lavorano con minore intensità in altre zone, ma nessuna di esse sarà disconnessa.

Gli scienziati suddividono le onde in 5 tipi, che corrispondono a cinque fasce di frequenza diverse. **Onde Gamma** (superiori ai 40 Hz), **onde Beta** (tra 40 – 13 Hz), **onde Alfa** (tra i 12.9 – 8 Hz), **onde Theta** (tra i 7.9 – 4 Hz) e **onde Delta** (tra i 3.9– 0.1 Hz).

Il cervello non percepisce frequenze sotto i 20-30 Hz (definite quindi frequenze infra-soniche). Ecco che vengono in aiuto i toni binaurali. Quindi, grazie al fenomeno della risonanza, se ascolto 1000 Hz da un auricolare e 980 Hz dall'altro, il cervello creerà un terzo suono (che non esiste, ma lui lo crea) di 20 Hz. In questo modo, con 20 Hz, andrò a stimolare le onde Beta. Se voglio stimolare la meditazione, ascolterò dei toni binaurali, ad esempio, che mi generano onde Alfa. La verità è che non ci sono onde cerebrali migliori o più speciali di altre. Sono tutte importanti, perché sono il risultato dell'attività elettrica dei nostri neuroni e di ciascuno dei nostri stati mentali.

Attenzione: anche se la differenza delle frequenze che ascoltiamo è pari a 5 Hz (1000 Hz sinistra – 995 Hz destra), quindi stimola le onde Theta, non raggiungiamo le condizioni che determinano queste onde. Quindi non basta ascoltare i suoni binaurali per addormentarsi. Tuttavia possiamo però utilizzare questi suoni per arrivare ad un buono stato di coscienza.

Elenco un link con toni bineurali www.martinadesimone.com

Capitolo 5

BIOHACKING ALIMENTAZIONE

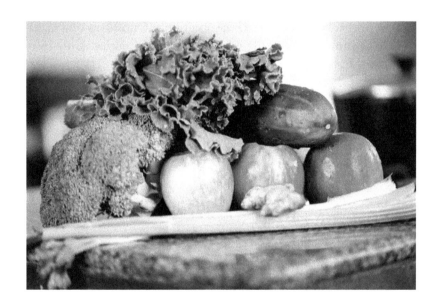

Alimentazione

- **Caffè**

Un buon hack è quello di assumere **caffè di buona qualità** (basso livello di micotossine) nel momento giusto. **Assumerlo la mattina appena alzato** (questo perché aumenta il metabolismo e le prestazioni mentali). Non berlo né in tarda giornata (per non disturbare il sonno.) e né in sovrabbondanza (per non sovra-stimolare la produzione di cortisolo).

Se non sopporti la caffeina, puoi assumere polifenoli con una tazza di the verde oppure una tazza di acqua, digiunando per minimo 16 ore, facendo così il digiuno intermittente (vedi dopo).

Si consiglia di non superare i 5 milligrammi / kilo. Per un uomo di 70 kg sono 350 milligrammi di caffeina (3/4 caffè espressi).

- Totale esclusione di cibo industriale.

- Riduci i carboidrati

- Consumare cibo organico e fresco il più possibile.

- Fare il pieno di antiossidanti con gli alimenti come frutta di bosco e verdura a km 0.

- Verdure preferibilmente crude. Sempre km 0.

- Evitare tutto ciò che può causare permeabilità intestinale (cereali, glutine, latticini, legumi, alcuni farmaci, spezie come il peperoncino/pepe e cibo industriale).

Il fenomeno della "permeabilità intestinale" prevede che, quando le giunture dei villi intestinali che proteggono l'intestino da schifezze (sostanze nocive, batteri, virus ecc.) si rompono, iniziano ad entrare sostanze indesiderati. L'intestino diventa permeabile, che porta a problemi e malattie.

• Usare grassi di qualità. Quindi mangiare carne allevata al pascolo e grassi da sego. Anche l'olio di cocco fa molto bene al nostro organismo.

• Spezie e cibi salutari possono essere: cannella, curcuma, zenzero, succo di lime dolce, aceto di mele, olio di senape, pompelmo, aglio, mirtilli, cioccolato fondente, broccoli, patate dolci, spinaci, papaya, the verde, peperone rosso.

Hack Digiuno

Cos'è il digiuno?

Per digiuno si intende un arco di tempo di "non alimentazione" di durata minima di 10 ore. Perché 10 ore? Perché a partire da 10 ore cominciano a manifestarsi quei meccanismi associati proprio al periodo di non alimentazione. Meno di 10 ore possiamo chiamarlo "pasto ritardato". In natura è facile che un animale rimanga a digiuno, specialmente carnivori (mangiano pochi pasti e abbondanti, ma non tutti i giorni).

Perché alcune volte, anche se non si mangia per ore, non si sente il bisogno di mangiare e altre volte anche passare 2 ore, abbiamo fame? Dipende dalla condizione di quel momento e dalla nostra alimentazione.

Benefici digiuno:

- **Aumento dei livelli dell'ormone della crescita.** Perché succede questo? Perché durante il digiuno il nostro corpo aumenta i livelli dell'ormone della crescita? Per la funzione che ha l'ormone della crescita nel nostro organismo. L'ormone della crescita, oltre a servire alla crescita tessuti, aumento massa muscolare o diminuire grasso corporeo, serve anche da ormone che regolarizza il metabolismo e glicemia (infatti l'ormone della crescita è iperglicemizzante). Cosa succede quando stiamo parecchie ore senza mangiare? Sta calando la glicemia, e quindi sopraggiunge il senso di fame e necessità di mangiare.

Quindi mantiene costante la glicemia e alza gli zuccheri nel sangue facendo risparmiare al corpo carboidrati che abbiamo di riserva e proteine che abbiamo a disposizione. È come se dicesse al corpo di conservare proteine e carboidrati, facendogli bruciare i grassi.

- **C'è una disintossicazione del corpo.** Non avendo cibo nel corpo, l'organismo ha modo di purificarsi.

- **Diminuiscono i livelli di insulina e dell'IGF-1** (somatomedina o Fattore di crescita insulino- simile).

L'IGF-1: si tratta di uno dei mediatori dell'ormone della crescita (GH) e serve quindi a stimolare lo sviluppo di alcuni tessuti del corpo umano, come le ossa, i muscoli, la pelle e il cervello.
L'IGF 1 è molto basso nel feto, ma in seguito comincia a crescere fino a raggiungere il suo picco massimo nella pubertà. Resta stabile per circa 40 anni, poi torna a decrescere con l'avanzare degli anni.
Una carenza di IGF1 può portare a disturbi della crescita (nanismo, gigantismo, bassa statura).

- **Aiuta l'autofagia.**

- **Aumenta la sensibilità all'insulina.**

- **Migliora il sistema immunitario.**

- **Migliora l'efficienza dei mitocondri** (anche grazie all'autofagia).

- **Avviene la lipolisi**: durante il digiuno il nostro corpo attinge prevalentemente dai grassi.

- **Si migliora l'assorbimento dei nutrienti.**

- **Si riassesta l'organismo.**

- **Avviene la chetosi** (il corpo per bruciare grassi avvia il processo di chetosi).

- **Miglioramento parametri ematici** (diminuzione colesterolo, si abbassa la glicemia, diminuisce la pressione sangue).

- **Diminuzione del livello di infiammazione.**

Tipi di digiuno

1. 10 ore di digiuno (mangiare ogni 10 ore).

2. Mangiare a colazione e cena, saltando il pranzo (16/8).

3. 16/8: si salta la colazione e si pranza e cena.

4. 1 pasto al giorno in qualsiasi momento.

5. Digiuno depurativo di più giorni, massimo 5.

Per chi non è adatto il digiuno?

-      Per chi segue diete ricche di carboidrati.
-      Per quelli che provano un forte senso di fame che non li fa concentrare.
-      Per chi si trova in uno stato non ottimale e debolezza generale di salute (ad esempio dopo un intervento chirurgico).
-      Per chi è sottopeso.
-      Chi non si sa ancora ascoltare il proprio corpo.
-      Se si hanno carenze e la dieta non è sufficientemente nutriente.

Quindi se hai delle carenze il digiuno è sconsigliato. Se provi a far digiuno hai un forte senso di fame, fatica a concentrarsi... Non farlo!

Hack Integrazione

Vediamo ora una serie di integratori che possono potenziare l'attività cognitiva, fisica e muscolare.

Vediamo cosa serve per vantaggi e benefici:

- **Vitamina D**: dose standard 5000 unità (verifica con analisi del sangue su parametro 25 OH- D che dev'essere compreso tra 70 e 90 ng/ml e paratormore (PTH) che dev'essere compreso tra 15-20 pg/ml).

La vitamina D viene prodotta anche esponendoci al sole che è quella fondamentale. Quindi è utile integrarla, ma stare al sole è fondamentale.

- **Vitamina A**: in forma naturale estratta dall'olio di fegato di merluzzo (o mangiare fegato).

- **Omega 3:**
Se nonostante seguiamo l'alimentazione corretta e vediamo che abbiamo problemi di concentrazione, apatia, dolori articolari, gengive che sanguinano, debolezza ecc. possiamo integrare essa con omega 3.

- **Vitamina C**: 1 grammo la mattina con colazione. È antiossidante per il corpo.

CONCLUSIONE

Spero che questo libro aiuti il maggior numero di persone non solo a liberarsi dal loro disturbo, ma anche a cambiare radicalmente la qualità della vita e l'aspettativa di vita.

Spero anche che se le persone con una formazione medica leggono questo libro, non lo giudicheranno.

Visto che siamo arrivati alla fine di questo libro, spero abbiate colto informazioni sane e preziose. Come abbiamo visto, gli effetti della temperatura fredda possono essere molto benefici per la salute. I mitocondri, che sono delle vere e proprie centrali di energia, vanno aiutati e potenziati, e quindi vanno hackerati. Con mitocondri poco funzionali, anche le nostre capacità fisiche e mentali si ridurranno notevolmente.

Abbiamo anche visto il tipo di alimentazione che ognuno di noi dovrebbe seguire, evitando ed eliminando cibi in scatola, prodotti da forno, olio fritto ecc.

Anche l'integrazione è molto importante, ma non dovrebbe essere sostituita dal pasto tradizionale.

Spero che applicherai questi preziosi consigli da domani, e non ci metterai molto a notare i primi risultati. Non sto dicendo che queste pratiche funzionano. Potrebbero essere semplicemente parole mie. Ti dico solo "sperimenta, sperimenta e sperimenta"!

Se questo libro ti è piaciuto, sarò molto contento sapere cosa hai apprezzato di più attraverso una piccola recensione direttamente su Amazon. Grazie!

WHAT LIES IN PARADISE

LEAH CUPPS

VISION FORTY

STAY IN THE KNOW

What's coming next from author Leah Cupps?

Get on the list to found out about upcoming book releases, bargains, giveaways and more.

www.leahcupps.com

To my parents, who taught me to love reading.

*To my husband, who endlessly inspires me
and puts up with my obsessive need to write.*

PROLOGUE

THE CIRCULAR STEEL barrel of a Glock nine-millimeter pushed roughly against Sydney's left temple. The gun was searing her skin, still warm from the last bullet fired. One large, tan, muscular arm wrapped around her neck, threatening to snuff out her last few breaths.

I should have seen this coming, she thought. *I should have known that if I agreed to go along with this ridiculous plan, something terrible would happen and I'd end up dead.*

A series of images from her life began to scroll across her brain, like the snapshots from her Instagram feed. She in pigtails blowing out the candles for her sixth birthday. The fabulous pink satin dress that peeked out from her graduation gown, bright enough to match to her beaming smile. A picture of her at a café in Paris posing with a freshly baked chocolate croissant and a steaming cappuccino. She could see the images, but all she could think about were the choices she didn't make and the people she neglected.

If she survived this moment, gun pressed against her temple, maybe she would start spending more time with her head in the real world, where life was messy and not one picture-perfect square after another. That was her mistake: projecting the perfect life made her believe she had the perfect life, but she didn't. Had she tapped the Do Not Disturb button every once in a while, maybe she would have sensed the lies that had begun to weave their way into the real world around her. She could have fallen in love with someone different, someone who led a simple, boring life, like an accountant or a mechanic. But who was she kidding? Love doesn't work that way.

Although there was shouting next to her ear, the voices sounded far away. All Sydney could hear was the blood thumping through her head and the *whoosh-whoosh* of her heart beating. The large tropical bushes that lined the walkway reached up toward the sky and bent down to form a canopy over the four of them, giving them respite from the burning Jamaican sun. She was not alone, but that didn't make the situation any better.

She could still hear the soft call of the ocean behind her but all she could see were palm leaves and the crushed gravel pathway beneath her. Sweat was pouring down her face, neck, and back, soaking the pale blue chiffon dress she had just posted herself wearing on social media a few hours ago.

If only my followers could see me now, Sydney thought.

She heard the click of the pistol's slide, chambering a round. Sydney didn't believe in bad luck, but this situation might surely change her mind. *Why me?* she thought as the world started to blur around her like a watercolor painting. She began to taste the tangy bit of blood forming at the back of her mouth. He was holding on too tightly. If only she could wake up from this nightmare and be somewhere else. Like when she woke up at the airport.

That was the beginning.

ONE

SYDNEY

SYDNEY EVANS HAD NEVER BEEN one for prescription medication. She rarely had headaches and managed to evade the flu virus year after year. In her early twenties she had her wisdom teeth pulled. Her dentist at the time had insisted on a prescription pain medication, which she took dutifully. It didn't agree with her. She fainted while trying to make the trip from the bathroom to the bed, woken only by the feeling of her cat Marlie's delicate tongue licking her face. That was the end of Sydney and little pills.

But lately, as the headaches became more frequent and the anxiety more intense, she realized she needed help to keep up with her life. Especially today, as she boarded a plane for the first time in six months. It seemed logical that she take a little something to help her relax. Well, she wanted more than to just relax. Perhaps *knocked out* was a better term. Plane rides had gone from a source of pleasure to a source of pain.

She had never taken Ambien before, though many friends had recommended it to her during the endless insomnia she experienced after Jack died. She had been able to squeeze in a last-minute appointment with Dr. Salinger, her general practitioner, to plead her case. He sat across from her in his drab ten-by-ten-foot exam room and quietly listened to her explain why she needed the drug. After a few minutes, he held up one of his long, clean hands and motioned for her to stop talking. He was happy to provide her with the prescription, but it came with a stern warning. He said there were a few serious possible side effects, including blackouts and amnesia. She had quickly brushed him off. "I have a few memories I'd like to forget," she joked. Dr. Salinger remained stoic in his response: "This is not something to be taken likely, Mrs. Evans."

As the passengers of the plane buzzed around her, Sydney reached down and pulled her vintage Louis Vuitton fringed crossover bag out from under her seat. She quickly unzipped the top and thrust her hand down into the bag, which was jammed full of her must-have travel supplies. She made a mental note to dump out the contents when she arrived at the hotel and do a snappy little post about what she had traveled with.

After about thirty seconds of rummaging around, she pulled out a small white pill bottle. She fumbled with the bottle cap, squeezed it open, and dropped a small pink pill into the palm of her hand. She paused and stared at her left hand. She could still see the tan line circling her ring finger, but there was no longer a ring there. Even though she had only been married for a short time, the lack of a wedding ring felt wrong to her. As if something was constantly missing from her hand. It was the first time she had ventured out sans wedding ring. Even though she had a variety of thin gold and silver bands sparkling on her other fingers, she still missed that ring the most.

Sydney sighed. *It's time to move on.* She pulled out a

bottle of FIJI water and one gulp later, the little magic pill slid down her throat. Surely this would make her plane ride a breeze. At least she could hope.

Around her, passengers were settling in as the plane rumbled forward on the tarmac. A dad with his towheaded daughters fumbled through his backpack to retrieve their iPads. "Daddy we want a show!" they cried over and over again. Sydney thought about how adorable they were, how she would love to have a few children herself one day.

She had grabbed an aisle seat, the large plane seating three on each side of the central walkway. Just to her left was a young couple, practically beaming with the newlywed glow. From what she could tell, they appeared to be maybe in their midtwenties. He had thick tortoise-shell glasses a hipster would wear and a hard part in his hair. She had shoulder-length, glossy black hair with purple highlights. They were casually dressed in hoodies, their backpacks stashed underneath the seat back in front of them. Out of the corner of her eye, she watched them flip through their wedding photos. Sydney felt a pang of sorrow mixed with envy.

She shifted her gaze to the guy in front of her, who swiped through the movie options on his television monitor. He seemed listless and unamused. Here was someone she could relate to. She had spent many nights over the last few months scrolling through her television guide. If she could lock onto a binge-worthy show, she'd have a few hours to escape from reality. Everywhere she looked there seemed to be a reminder of what her life could have been, what it is now, and what it wasn't.

Sydney strapped on her noise-canceling headset and tuned in to her meditation app. Another suggestion from a friend: guided meditation. As sounds of the ocean mixed with flutes and wind chimes streamed into her ear drums, she let herself think about the upcoming few days.

She was headed to the wedding of the year, the marriage of debutante Marissa Schumacher and her dashing fiancé, Ethan Evans. Marissa was her best friend since college, a friendship that was thirteen years strong. Her fiancé was Sydney's former brother in law, Jack's identical twin. Seeing the identical twin brother of your dead husband get married was certainly not something your average person had to face. And it was with great difficulty that she had even agreed to go to the wedding. To be frank, she wanted to wipe the entire past year from her memory. She knew that one day the events of this year would feel like a distant memory and all the pain it caused would collapse into a dull ache. But she had promised her best friend that she would be there. Sydney was a loyal friend, and this was the biggest day of Marissa's life.

Marissa and Ethan's swanky nuptials were to take place on the idyllic white beaches of Jamaica. Several local media magazines from Chicago were flying in to cover the glamorous production. Marissa herself had spent little time planning the event, leaving all the details to a well-known wedding planner named Jessica Gaines. Jessica was known for creating over-the-top events with a price tag to match. Sydney was sure that no expense would be spared in creating a magical, unforgettable experience for everyone who attended. She had searched the hotel website, scouting for spots to shoot her own outfits, and the hotel just oozed glamour and prestige.

As for being maid of honor, Sydney had it easy. All she had to do was show up. Marissa had made it clear to the planner that under no circumstances would Sydney be required to do anything but be there for the wedding.

Marissa had graciously left all the maid of honor duties to their other best friend, Elizabeth Ortez. Lizzy, as they affectionately called her, was their college roommate from sophomore year and a dedicated friend. It was apparent to anyone who knew them that Lizzy simply adored Marissa and Sydney.

With Lizzy at the helm of the bachelorette party and bridal shower, Sydney could relax and try to focus on making it through the entire ordeal without having a complete meltdown. She didn't like to admit to anyone how hard the last few months had been. She had showed up at events with her photographer, Manuel, in tow and he snapped pictures of each soiree with glee. Her followers had been especially responsive and cheered Sydney on as she moved forward with her life. She had to admit, from the outside, it seemed like her life had pretty much gone on without a hitch. But all the pain was just below the surface. She pushed those thoughts to the back of her mind and refocused on the upcoming wedding.

As a seasoned traveler, Sydney had been to many islands in the Caribbean but never Jamaica. She was partially looking forward to a change of scenery and the chance to explore a new place that had no memories tied to her past. The thought of the sand bubbling up between her toes and the feeling of the hot sun hitting her freshly spray-tanned skin sounded almost enjoyable to her.

At least all of her 416,000 followers on Instagram would find her trip enviable. Keeping up her social media feed was validation of her successful transition from happy wife to content single woman. The thought of her followers made her almost subconsciously reach for her phone. The sleek iPhone X with its clear acrylic case and Swarovski crystal design felt like home. Just the weight of it in her hand seemed to release some kind of positive chemical response in her brain. She abandoned the soothing sounds of her meditation app and began an endless scroll through all the likes, comments, and tags on her Instagram feed.

Over the last four years, she had delivered a pretty white smile and a fabulous string of carefully crafted outfits. A colorful display of Sydney's creative vision for her life. She hadn't sought a career as a professional influencer; it just sort of fell into her carefully styled lap. Makeup and fashion had always been a hobby for Sydney, and when she started posting photos of her everyday outfits, the response had been immediate and positive. Over a few short years, she had built her following from a few hundred friends to several hundred thousand eager fans. The brand partnerships she had developed as well as the steady income from clothing affiliate sales had allowed her to quit her job at a marketing firm and pursue her career online full time.

She hadn't slowed down since her husband died, and Marissa's wedding was just another mountain she was determined to climb. Sydney had meticulously packed her bags with just the right collection of resort wear, from beach hats and long caftans to bright lace-up espadrilles and mirrored sunglasses. She had multiple camera lenses, a tripod, and other equipment packed away and ready to make the ideal shot.

Letting her audience down equaled failure and meant facing the fact that maybe life wasn't so perfect after all. They had all reveled at her strength after her husband's death and cheered her resilience as a young widow. The comments and messages had come streaming in day after day, giving Sydney a sense of community and comfort, even though they were people she had never met and would likely never share a coffee with.

The death of Jack Evans. It had been six months. Mornings without him were still the hardest. She would wake up, reach her hands across the smooth white sheets of her unmade bed, and search for the warmth of his skin. She wondered when she would stop reaching out and coming up empty-handed.

She missed him. She wondered if that would ever go away. The ache of losing someone you thought would be by your side for life. It pained her to think of the weeks leading up to his death, which were peppered with petty fights and contempt.

Jack had all the trappings of the perfect husband: smart and successful, plus good-looking enough to cause women to stare at him from across a restaurant. He seemed perpetually fit, with a full head of warm-brown hair that had a carefully styled wave to it. Unlike his clean-shaven brother, Jack kept a neatly trimmed beard that bordered on a five o'clock shadow. He had a slight hook in his nose that when he was tan made him look a bit like a Greek god. He was thoughtful, punctual, even stylish. He never left the toilet seat up. They made a fantastic-looking couple, picture-perfect. Although much to her disappointment, they rarely took photographs together.

But there was something about him, a small part he kept hidden. Perhaps it was the way he snapped upright when she walked into his office or the vague answers he gave her after he returned from a business trip. As the co-founder of DoubleDownCasino.com, she knew he had a lot of responsibilities that ranged from his coding and developing to hiring and managing staff. Jack was adamant about keeping his business separate from his personal life, so Sydney didn't poke or pry too much at home. The sex was great, even if they didn't talk much anymore. That still makes for a good marriage, right? She realized later, their union was built on a foundation striped with fault lines. It only took small earthquakes for those cracks to become divides. She felt her heart begin to ache again.

No, she told herself, *don't go there. Look ahead.*

She did look ahead, right at the flight attendant who was standing over her with a wide grin and brassy blond curls that dusted her shoulders.

"Excuse me, ma'am, may I have a glass of champagne?"

"Right away," she said with a smile. It was Sydney's inaugural voyage into first class, and so far, everything was living up to the hype. The seats were more comfortable. The leg room was spacious. The service was quick. Even with her success as an influencer, Sydney felt some things were too extravagant. But Marissa had insisted on paying for her first-class seat. She switched her phone over to selfie mode and quickly snapped a photo, later captioning it "First-class virgin no more." She stared for a moment at her own image: artfully filled-in eyebrows and long, full eyelashes framing deep-green eyes. She had a petite nose with a round tip that she carefully contoured to make it look longer and narrower. Her lips were a fully plumped shade of pink, a combination of lip fillers and pink liner she used to enhance her natural pout. Her blond hair fell in long waves that nearly hit her waist, compliments of her freshly applied hair extensions. She sighed. It was a perfectly executed look, even if some days she didn't feel like it looked like her. She hit Post and her first-class photo went live on her feed. The wine arrived just a few minutes later.

As she stared down the glass, she wondered if it was a good idea to mix prescription medication with alcohol. Probably not. But she didn't feel up to making responsible decisions today. She felt the bubbles fizz and pop against her nose, and she tipped the glass, perfectly chilled wine sliding easily down her throat.

The lights in the cabin dimmed, the plane pushed forward, and she suddenly felt drowsy, like a baby being cradled to sleep. Sydney kept herself awake just long enough to stash her phone in her designer bag, snap on her velvety pink neck pillow, and recline her seat. Her last thoughts were of palms trees swaying high above her as the warm breezes of Jamaica greeted her with a salty kiss. The curved walls of the plane cabin turned to black.

SYDNEY HEARD A DEEP, throaty voice saying her name repeatedly as her eyes began to flutter open. The room she was in was a series of black and grey blobs that slowly came into focus. As she peeled her skin away from the cold laminate table top, she wiped the drool dripping out the side of her mouth. She reached up and pulled the hair from her eyes. Her head felt heavy as she sat upright. A sterile grey room came into focus.

One particular large blob was forming into a large man, who was wearing a slight scowl on his face. He was sitting across from her, dressed in a black uniform with a patch on the front that read U.S. Department of Homeland Security. Sydney blinked several times. *This can't be good*, she thought.

"Good morning, Mrs. Evans," he said with a gruff voice that rattled when he spoke. "Glad to have you back with us. My name is Inspector Sam O'Connell. I'd like to ask you a few questions."

TWO

ETHAN

ETHAN EVANS LEANED back into the plush cream uphol-stery of the Bombardier jet and peered out the oval window next to his seat. He rubbed his palms along the polished wood armrests and then ran a hand through his thick brown hair. The stewardess, Jackie, had just delivered a much-needed beverage. She was a severe-looking woman, rail thin with a sharp bob that floated just above her shoulders. Her thick black glasses reminded him of his high school librar-ian, who had frequently swatted him with a wooden ruler for snickering during study hall.

A small cocktail napkin sat squarely underneath the scotch in front him, soaking up the condensation from his glass. The Glenlivet Single Malt scotch had slid down his throat a little too quickly. Now he sat back, letting the gentle release of the alcohol fall over him like a warm bath. He could see the Schumacher Oil logo emblazoned on the side, with the letters S and O intertwined. He stared out the window again as the beads of water slid down the side of the crystal glass and tried to enjoy his plush surroundings.

Being involved with someone of Marissa Schumacher's

wealth and stature certainly had its benefits, including the luxury private jet he was currently lounging in. He could see her long tan legs peeking out from the cockpit as she led her friend Lizzy Ortez and Lizzy's boyfriend, Will Sauder, on a tour of the plane. Marissa was the heiress apparent of a sprawling oil fortune her great-grandparents had begun to amass several decades ago. Schumacher Oil had been a family tradition going back three generations. Their holdings began in the oil industry and quickly expanded into a variety of global ventures, including wireless technology, bio technology, and agriculture, with some of the biggest names in each respective industry. With offices and employees across the globe, the publicly traded company was known worldwide. But the majority of the stock still remained within the original Schumacher family. That lineage had ended with Marissa. Her inheritance came much sooner than the world had expected when her parents both died while flying through a storm in their private jet, during her junior year in college. He shuddered when he thought of their demise, as the similarity of the situation was not lost on him. He liked to keep his head clear, but this flight might require another scotch.

Lucky for Marissa, who was only twenty-one at the time of their death, the management team who was in place did a fantastic job of keeping the company barreling forward. Marissa had hardly set foot in the corporate headquarters. Instead she lived off the dividends of her vast estate.

It had been about a year and a half since he and Marissa had met. All the events in his life seemed to have been stuck in fast forward since then. He had been immediately attracted to her, as any man would. She was tall, with a fit physique from years of Pilates and playing tennis. Her sparkling blue eyes popped against the dark auburn hair that framed her heart-shaped face. But what kept him interested wasn't her looks or the vast fortune she had inherited. He had dated his share of heiresses and beautiful women. It was the fact that his twin, Jack, was head over heels for her best friend Sydney.

They had all met the same night, and he knew his brother well enough to know that Sydney had immediately stolen his heart. Jack became obsessed with her. He spent every spare moment he could following her around Chicago and across the world, taking photos for her Instagram page and catering to her every need. It was then that Ethan felt Jack pull away from him for the first time in his life. They had rarely been separated since birth—even during college and their years living the bachelor lifestyle, they stuck together. When Jack began to prioritize his relationship with Sydney over his own brother, Ethan decided it was time that maybe he settle down as well. And it didn't hurt that Marissa's fortune came along with the package.

Ethan and Marissa had bounced around the United States and Europe flying first class, but the Schumacher jet was reserved for special occasions. Their upcoming nuptials on the silky white beaches of Jamaica certainly qualified. Flying by private jet was one of the many luxuries that Marissa seemed to take for granted. He couldn't blame her; she had known nothing else.

Still, Ethan couldn't help but envy her for the ease and freedom with which she experienced the world. Not only had all of her needs been met since the day she was born, her desires had been met as well. Ethan and Jack, on the other hand, had been born into an unstable household. Their parents not only struggled financially, but mentally and emotionally as well. They battled alcohol and drug abuse, which often affected their ability to hold steady jobs or keep up with rent. It certainly made parenting their energetic young twin boys a challenge.

He jiggled the ice in his glass and thought about the past. For the brothers it had been a life of feast or famine. Highs and lows. Whenever his dad got a new job, the family would all go out to a nice dinner. His mother would put on a pretty blue dress she reserved for special occasions. It had a Peter Pan collar and delicate lace detailing that ran across the front. She would nervously finger the lace as they waited for the hostess to find them a table. The boys in their button-down shirts would stand quietly behind her, afraid to move a muscle and thus invite the wrath of their father. The meal would begin with their father telling jokes and chatting with the boys about school. His mother would smile silently and seemed to soak up the moment as a glass of wine dangled in her hand. On the outside their family looked nearly perfect.

But after two, three, or even four drinks at the restaurant, his parents would almost always get in a fight. Usually because his dad thought someone was hitting on his mother. A loud argument followed, and they would inevitably be asked to leave. Holidays were equally as unpredictable. One year the living room was so packed full of gifts on Christmas morning, you could barely find a space to sit. His mother and father had been waiting downstairs for the boys to wake up, beaming with pride as they ripped through one treasure after another. The following year, the boys were greeted with solemn looks from their parents, as they sat on the couch with a half-empty bottle of whiskey between them. The doorbell rang around noon that year, and a local charity organization dropped off a meal for their family. His father was furious with his mother for reaching out for help. And by the sounds that came from the bedroom that evening, they knew she had paid for her mistake.

There was an upside to his tumultuous upbringing, however. Ethan and his brother, Jack, developed a toughness and self-reliance you didn't have when there was a silver spoon in your mouth. Whether it was finding food or escaping the beatings of their father, being clever and likable was a sure way to survive. It was comforting to know what he was made of, but Ethan never wanted to go back to that life again. The struggles that he experienced as a child powered his inner drive to succeed and leave that life as far behind him as possible.

"Not a bad way to fly, man. Thanks for the ride," Will said as he flopped down into the seat across from Ethan. His shrill voice, which always sounded as if he were a cheap car salesman, cut through Ethan's thoughts. He leaned forward, holding his matching glass forward as an offer to toast.

Will was average in every way, from his sand-colored hair to his muddy-brown eyes and pale complexion. He seemed to have a vast collection of performance knit polos, which he paired with plain black pants and black loafers. Aside from the shoes, he appeared to be ready to golf at any moment. But what Will lacked in style, he certainly made up for in his relentless enthusiasm to land Ethan as a client.

"Glad to have you with us," Ethan said, clinking his glass against Will's and forcing a smile. Will and Lizzy had essentially invited themselves along for the ride. Lizzy had a knack for cashing in favors. She had recently lost her job as a private school teacher and, as a favor to Marissa, he hired her to work in his office. Alice Mitchell, his secretary, had quickly put her to work running errands, answering the phones, and picking up lunches for his staff.

Although Ethan felt he had paid her handsomely, Lizzy

mentioned to Marissa that it would be difficult for her to afford a ticket down to Jamaica. Instead of just buying her a ticket on a commercial plane, Marissa had generously offered to fly her and Will down on the private jet, much to Ethan's chagrin. He was looking forward to some quiet time.

"So, Ethan, I have been wanting to ask you." Ethan felt his teeth clench as he waited for what he knew was coming next. "Have you been getting my messages about having a lunch at your office? You know, a chance for me to introduce myself to your staff?"

Ethan tried to hide the grimace on his face. Will had recently launched a career selling life insurance and was ever eager to build up his portfolio of clients. Ethan had to tip his hat to the relentless approach with which he sought out new customers. However, there was zero chance Will would ever land him as a client. "Oh yes, Will, I apologize. Work has been really busy. I just haven't had a chance to look at our office calendar."

"Oh sure, sure. No problem. How about Monday August 24? Isn't that when you get back from the honeymoon?" Ethan tried to find a quick excuse. Nothing came to mind quickly enough, so he finally conceded.

"That sounds fine. Why don't you call my secretary, Alice, and she can set something up?"

Ethan heard some soft giggling as Marissa and Lizzy walked up to their seats from the back of the plane. The jet could hold up to sixteen people and included a small kitchen and quiet suite in the back.

"You boys talking business?" Lizzy said as she plopped down into her seat across the aisle. "Busy Lizzy," as Marissa and Sydney liked to call her, was a short, round Hispanic woman with black ringlets that danced around her round face. She was pretty with her olive skin, full lips, and almond-shaped brown eyes. Ethan always thought she'd be a knockout if she dropped about twenty pounds. But Lizzy was happily plump and seemed to live in a world where Taco Tuesday and *Game of Thrones* outweighed a diet or a trip to the gym. At the moment, she was carrying a small wineglass that sparkled with champagne.

"Ethan just invited me to host a lunch at his office," Will responded with a smile from ear to ear.

"Oh, did he?" Marissa walked up to Ethan's seat and gently sat down in his lap, wrapping one arm around his neck. She gave him a small kiss on the lips and then pulled back to look at him with a rueful smile. "That's so nice of you, darling."

Marissa knew better than anyone what it was like to have everyone asking you for a favor.

"Well, I just gave Lizzy a tour of the plane, and now I think it's time I have a drink." She turned her gaze across the aisle. "Lizzy, would you like another glass of champagne?"

"Please," she said with a smile.

Marissa rose from Ethan's lap and headed back toward the kitchen. Ethan looked down at his phone, scrolling through emails to avoid eye contact with Will. He seemed to take the hint and jumped across the aisle to sit closer to Lizzy. Marissa returned a few moments later with a jiggling glass of what he guessed was a vodka and tonic. She handed him another scotch.

As the drinks flowed, the four of them shared stories of their travels. Some of the predicaments Will had found himself in were quite funny, while Marissa and Lizzy shared a lot of history traveling during college. About an hour later, Lizzy grew quiet.

"Marissa, I think I must have had a little too much. I'm not feeling well." Lizzy placed a hand on her stomach, emphasizing her point. He could see some of the color had drained from her typically rosy cheeks, and yet a sheen of sweat glistened under the cabin lights. "Would you mind if I laid down in the back?"

"Of course." Marissa stood up and walked over to her friend. "Come on, I'll get you settled. I need my bridesmaid in top form for the wedding." Lizzy stumbled a bit as she stood up. Marissa grabbed her elbow and steadied her as they headed toward the back of the plane. She looked over her shoulder and gave a knowing look to Ethan. Lizzy had a reputation for overindulging.

After Lizzy had gone to sleep, the plane grew quiet. Each of the remaining passengers in the main cabin retreated back into their phones. An hour passed. The pilot's voice broke the silence, announcing that landing in Jamaica was imminent.

Marissa looked up from her phone at Ethan. "I'll wake up Lizzy."

As she stood up and made her way back to the rear cabin, Ethan couldn't help but admire his soon to be wife. She was beautiful to look at, as anyone could see. But she also had a certain dignified grace about her that made him admire her on a deeper level. Truthfully, he knew he had found the perfect woman. No one would ever match her in his eyes.

He felt the plane dip slightly as they prepared for landing. As he buckled his seatbelt and leaned back into his chair, he heard Marissa's voice softly calling for Lizzy. Then her tone seemed to change, and her voice began to rise. Ethan felt nerves under his skin prickle.

"Ethan! Will! Come quick," Marissa suddenly shouted. "She's not breathing!"

Ethan and Will leapt out of their chairs in perfect sync

and ran to the back of the plane. When they burst through the cabin's partition, he could see Marissa hunched over Lizzy, frantically shaking her body. One of her tan, plump arms flopped over the side of the built-in sofa.

"I don't understand, she's not waking up!" she said turning her wide eyes toward him and Will. "Lizzy!" she said as she looked back toward her friend's still body. Lizzy's eyes were closed, and her mouth was parted slightly. Her lips were blue. Will leapt forward into action.

"I—I know CPR, let me see if I can help," he said bending down over Lizzy. He pressed both of his hands on her chest and began pumping them in a rhythmic motion. "Lizzy, honey, can you hear me?"

The next few minutes slogged on. Will seemed determined that his frantic motions were going to bring Lizzy out of her sleep. Her body remained still.

The plane descended below 10,000 feet. Ethan and Marissa stood side by side, completely motionless. As if the plane was still moving but their bodies were suspended in midair. Finally, Ethan couldn't take watching the awful scene any longer. He reached down and put a hand on Will's shoulder. The pumping stopped, and Will sat back on his heels. He was breathless. He pulled his hand back from her chest and slowly reached a shaky hand toward her neck. He pressed two fingers against the side of her neck and then slowly let his arm drop to his side. None of them said a word.

Jackie suddenly appeared at the partition opening, breaking the silence that held them captive. Her wide eyes betrayed her surprise.

"Mrs. Schumacher," she said, as she placed a hand on the wall to steady herself. "Please, I need everyone to take their seats, we will be landing soon."

No one moved. The plane forced them to bend their knees as they angled down, and that seemed to finally break their trance. Jackie stared at them, seemingly bewildered by their lack of cooperation. Then she followed their gazes down to the motionless body. "Is everything okay with Miss Ortez?"

Ethan raised his eyes from Lizzy and looked at the stewardess, feeling numb from shock. It took a moment for the words in his mind to travel down his brain and onto his lips.

"No, ma'am," he said, his hollow voice barely louder that the hum of the jet engines. "Miss Ortez is dead."

THREE
SYDNEY

SYDNEY WILLED her eyes to stay open, but her heavily enhanced lashes were threatening to close them once again. She glanced around the room and noticed a large grey door but no windows. Above her, a drop ceiling framed tacky florescent light panels that rained down cold blue light into the room. Two sturdy metal chairs sat on each side of a pale cream Formica table with stainless steel legs. The floors were laminate and provided no damper for any sound in the room, including the sound of a foot tapping on the floor.

The foot belonged to a large man who was sitting across from her. He loomed over her with all the intensity of a silverback gorilla. His forehead was scrunched down into his eyebrows, a look that suggested he was frustrated, and the tapping revealed his impatience. Behind him she could see a three-foot-wide mirror.

The scene felt weirdly familiar. About a year ago, when she was traveling back from Europe, Sydney had been detained for several hours because she took a photo while moving through Customs. She almost missed her connecting flight, and she nearly lost her phone to the

Customs and Border Protection police. She had spent at least an hour pent up in a room, just like the one she was in, babbling on about why she took the photo and what she did for a living. The lesson she learned in that situation: the less you say, the better.

Her first impulse was to reach down into her purse and grab her phone. Her lifeline. Sydney's phone held all the essential pieces of her life: family, friends, career. To be apart from it was virtual death. She slept with it by her bedside, kept it just outside the glass enclosure of her shower while she was bathing. She biked, hiked, ran with it close to her chest. It wasn't enough to just enjoy those things —they had to be documented on her various social media accounts. Photograph, filter, post, repeat. She always added a witty caption and a link to everything she was wearing.

What she saw, however, when she looked down at her side was an empty space. She stared for a moment, realizing that the clothes on her back were the only possessions she had with her. She returned her gaze to the gorilla-man, who looked increasingly impatient, and tucked a strand of artfully curled hair behind her ear.

"Have you seen my cell phone?" she asked.

"You will receive your belongings after we've had a chance to talk, Mrs. Evans." He leaned forward, causing the joints of his chair to shriek in response to his hefty frame. The sound was like a knife stabbing at the folds in her brain. Dark stubble on his round tan cheeks clung to his skin like a black cloud. His rumpled uniform fit him like a black trash bag, a little too tight in the chest and baggy in the arms. It looked as if he had attempted to control the black curls of his hair with petroleum jelly, as it glistened under the cold light in the room. "Now, are you ready to answer a few questions?"

Sydney reached a shaky hand forward to take the coffee. The steaming, tar-like liquid inside her cup was a far cry from her usual frothy cappuccino, but she took a swig and then a deep breath. The burnt smell reminded her of a gas station where they left the pots simmering too long. She felt uneasy and on edge, and her previous experience with Customs told her to tread carefully. She hadn't done anything wrong. *Or had she?* The details of the plane ride where not exactly clear yet.

"Um, yes I think so." The hot coffee seared her throat. "Where am I?"

"We are inside the Homeland Security section of the Atlanta airport. The plane you were on was diverted here. You were escorted off the plane." He paused, squinting at her. "Do you have any memory of leaving the plane?"

She smoothed out her eyebrows and rubbed her temples. The last memory she had was the delicious, bubbling glass of champagne sliding down her throat and then the sweet relief of sleep. She could feel a strong headache brewing.

"Um, no, I do not."

"I thought so," he said.

She could have sworn the right side of his mouth lifted in a bit of a smile. She got the feeling he knew something that she didn't. "Did you take something on the plane to help you sleep?"

Sydney felt her cheeks burn. *The sleeping pills!* She must have blacked out, just like the doctor warned her.

"Yes, I took Ambien. But I have a prescription. From my doctor." She emphasized the last three words.

"Indeed, you do. We found the bottle in your purse."

"You went through my purse?" The comment caught Sydney off guard. She knew she had certain rights when traveling, and rifling through her purse felt like a violation. "What is going on here? Why am I being detained?"

O'Connell cocked his massive head to one side, seemingly studying her from across the table. "Mrs. Evans, I promise to tell you everything you need to know. But I just need you to answer a few more questions first."

Sydney let a puff of air leave her throat to show her irritation. "Fine. What else do you need to know?"

"What is your relationship to Marissa Schumacher?"

"Marissa?" Her mind raced. *The wedding!* She was going to be late if she didn't get out of this tiny prison of a room and on the next flight ASAP. "Well, she's my best friend. In fact, I'm on my way to her wedding. Why?"

O'Connell ignored her question. "And Ethan Evans. What is your relationship with him?"

Sydney felt like someone had punched her in the gut. The words *brother-in-law* swept across her mind like a billboard. But she couldn't say it. It hurt to say it.

"He is Marissa's fiancé."

"I see," he said, keeping his gaze steadily focused on her. The intense staring made her uncomfortable. "And what about Elizabeth Ortez? Is she also a friend of yours?"

"Yes, she's my friend. The three of us went to college together."

"The three of you, as in Ethan and Marissa? Or Marissa and Elizabeth?"

Sydney, growing impatient, resisted the urge to roll her eyes dramatically. *Keep it simple.*

"Marissa, Elizabeth, and I," she said with all the patience she could muster.

"Right," he said as he reached down into the pocket of his polyester shirt and pulled out a pair of reading glasses. A plain-looking yellow folder sat in front of him. He flipped it open with a pudgy finger and inspected the pages inside.

"It says here you were on a direct flight from Chicago to Negril, Jamaica. Is that correct?"

"Yes."

"Why were you flying to Jamaica?"

"For a wedding."

"Whose wedding?"

"As I said before, Marissa and Ethan's wedding." She didn't try to hide the irritation in her voice.

"I see. How do you feel about your friend Marissa getting married?"

Sydney felt the heat rise in her cheeks again. "Well, that's none of your business." She leaned back into her chair and folded her arms across her chest.

O'Connell removed the glasses perched on his nose and folded his hands in front of him. For what seemed like an eternity, he simply stared at her. The last bit of patience Sydney was holding on to began to completely unravel. A headache elevated the situation.

"Mr. O'Connell, what is going on here? You pulled me off my flight, locked me in this room, and now you want to chit-chat about my circle of friends?" She could barely control the outrage now spewing from her vocal chords. "As I said, I am on my way to a wedding! A wedding I am going to miss if you don't let me get on the next flight as soon as possible."

"Mrs. Evans, this room is not locked. You are free to go whenever you like."

"Great. Fine." She stood up too quickly and nearly stumbled. She was still feeling a little shaky from her drug-and-wine-infused slumber. "I would like my things back, please," she said with as much confidence as she could muster. "And I will be on my way."

The sound of the chair screeching behind her reverberated throughout the room. Just as she was about to head for the door, O'Connell spoke again.

"But there is something you might want to know first."

She snapped her attention back to him.

"And what's that?" she said impatiently.

"You might want to sit down," he said and gestured to the chair she had just abandoned.

She glared down at him, the florescent panel lights illuminating specs of dust suspended in the air between them. "I'll stand."

O'Connell took a deep breath.

"Mrs. Evans, I regret to inform you that your friend Elizabeth Ortez is dead."

FOUR
SYDNEY

"LIZZY IS DEAD!?" It took a moment for the words to register in her mind. It was as if a giant vacuum had sucked the air out of the room. The dull ache in her head broke into a full-on storm of pain.

"What do you mean she is dead? How is that possible? I just talked to her an hour ago, well, I mean, texted. She sent me a message right before I boarded my flight."

The words seemed to flow from her mouth, undeterred by the alarm bells ringing in her brain.

"I'm sorry, Mrs. Evans. Lizzy became...suddenly ill on the plane."

The room blurred and Sydney's eyes began to swell with tears. She felt her body begin to give out and reached down to steady herself with the table. "Suddenly ill? And...then she died?"

"Yes, she was ill and then she died of cardiac arrest." He paused, taking a deep breath. "Mrs. Evans, we believe she was murdered." He waited for her to respond, but Sydney sat still holding her breath. He blinked at her and continued. "Poison was found in a glass of champagne she had been drinking on the plane. Marissa found her unresponsive in the back of the jet when they were about to land."

Sydney's hand shot up to her mouth, covering her lips in horror. *Poison?! Poor Lizzy!* The tears began to burst from her eyes as sobs exploded from her chest. Grief was not a revelation; she had been crying every day since Jack had left her. But Lizzy? She couldn't believe such a sweet soul would be murdered. *Who would want to hurt Lizzy?*

O'Connell's demeanor seemed to change when he saw how distraught she was from the news. The cold metal chair beneath her shuddered as she felt deep, heavy sobs shake her body. He quietly slid a pack of tissues over to her, which she grabbed up and quickly saturated with a mixture of tears and makeup.

After a few minutes of sobbing, Sydney tried to pull herself together. She took a couple of deep breaths, pulled her shoulders back, and faced her interrogator.

"Okay. I...Is this why I'm here?" A thought suddenly thundered into her mind, cutting through her thoughts of grief. "Do you think I had something to do with her death?"

"We are not making any assumptions at this point," he said, looking away and shifting slightly in his chair. "But any information you can provide would be extremely helpful."

Sydney wiped another mascara-filled tear from her face. She felt her grief give way to another emotion: anger.

"Of course. Anything I can do to help."

Inspector O'Connell took a deep breath that expanded his rib cage beyond its usual massive size. He began pelting her with a barrage of questions, which she barely remembered answering. He wanted to know how the three of them had met. How much time she had spent with Lizzy before the wedding. What their relationship had been like the last few months. It wasn't until he began to ask about Marissa and Lizzy, specifically, that she became concerned.

"Do you know of any reason why Marissa would want to hurt Lizzy?"

Sydney stared at him in disbelief. "No, of course not."

"What about Ethan—would he have any reason to want Lizzy...out of the picture?"

"No, we all loved Lizzy. She was sweet and caring." She felt her eyes sting with tears again. Her head seemed to be throbbing louder than anyone else in the room. But her outrage at Lizzy's death kept her focused.

"Did you know that Miss Ortez was working with Mr. Evans in his office?"

"Really? Uh...no. I didn't know that." She vaguely remembered something about Lizzy losing her job at a private prep school in Milwaukee. She had been so preoccupied with her work that she hadn't exactly been quick about returning Lizzy's calls.

"I thought she was one of your closest friends?"

"Well yes, but, I have been so busy with work." She sighed and looked at her hands, feeling the guilt seize her. "We haven't spoken much lately."

"I see. Well, do you think that Miss Ortez working in Mr. Evans' office would cause any trouble between him and Miss Schumacher? Would she be jealous?"

Sydney nearly spilled her coffee on the table. "No. Marissa has no reason to be jealous of Lizzy. That's crazy."

"And why is that, Mrs. Evans?"

"Marissa has it all. She is beautiful, wealthy, smart—and she is actually a good person. Lizzy has always struggled to find...stability. So no, it would be the other way around, if anything."

"Hmm. Okay."

She could see him scribbling down some notes on a small yellow pad lying next to the folder. Sydney craned her neck and tried to see what he was writing. She couldn't make anything out.

"What about Mr. Evans—do you think her working in his office would cause any problems? Problems that would—"

"Would make him want to kill Lizzy? That's a bit of a stretch, don't you think? He could have just fired her."

O'Connell studied her for a moment. She could see by the way his eyes moved around his face that he was thinking something but not telling her. Sydney knew people often underestimated her because of her looks, but her intuition had never failed her in situations like this one.

"Is there something you are not telling me, inspector?"

He leaned forward and put his massive elbows on the table. "Mrs. Evans, I assume you know the sensitive nature of Mr. Evans' online gambling business, especially given that your deceased husband was his partner?"

She gave a slight nod, fighting back the fireball of grief burning in the back of her throat.

He continued, "Do you think it's possible that Miss Ortez found something at his office, or in his files, that she wasn't supposed to find? Like a piece of evidence that might point to something illegal happening at DoubleDownCasino.com?"

Sydney swallowed deeply and considered what he was saying for a moment.

Of course, it was possible.

DoubleDownCasino.com had always operated in a legal grey area. Jack had assured her over and over again that it was a legal business and that the law was on their side. But she knew by the amount of stress that Jack was under that bounds of legality were being tested. Ethan was always a bit of a wild card. His brother, Jack, balanced him out with rational, responsible thinking. This caused a lot of tension between them. Tension that Sydney could see but that Jack refused to confide in her about. It created a small divide in their marriage that had widened over time.

But in this case, she had to protect Marissa and Ethan. The wedding meant so much to the both of them. She wanted to see them succeed as a couple, she needed them to succeed. It gave her a sliver of hope.

"Oh no, that's not possible," she said, regaining focus. "Everything in Ethan's business is completely aboveboard. He is in constant contact with his lawyer to make sure all the legalities are ironed out, before he does anything." *Technically that's not true*, she thought as the words fell out of her mouth. But O'Connell didn't need to know that.

She could see the shades of doubt cast across his face. She needed to redirect the conversation, and quickly.

"Have you spoken with Will?"

"Uh…" He looked down at his papers and began shuffling through them. "William Sauder?"

"Yes, Will is Lizzy's boyfriend. They've been living together for four years. She was always a little too good for him in my opinion, and he sells *life insurance* for a living."

Even as the words came out of her mouth, she found it hard to believe that Will would have anything to do with Lizzy's death. But she'd seen enough episodes of *Snapped* to know that life insurance policies were often a motive for murder. By the quizzical look on his face, she seemed to have caught the stalwart inspector off guard, which gave her a new wave of boldness.

"Hmm, we will take a look."

"Also, what about her cousin, Javier? He was always

asking her for money. I think he was involved with drugs. Would he benefit from her death?" She arched a carefully drawn eyebrow at him to emphasize her question. "That might be worth looking into."

She was on roll now, throwing out suspects like candy at a Fourth of July parade. O'Connell didn't look too convinced by any of her ideas, but at least it would spread his attention thin enough to maybe take some of the heat off of Marissa and Ethan.

O'Connell jotted down what she assumed was Javier's name on the notepad in front of him. He tapped the table a few times with his black ball point pen. "Mrs. Evans, as you know, we have your cell phone. As a courtesy, we'd like to ask your permission to search your phone for any evidence in the case."

Sydney's chest fluttered in a bit of a panic. *Search my phone? For evidence?* She couldn't for the life of her think of anything in her phone that would be related to Lizzy's killer. In fact, they'd likely find nothing but thousands of photos of herself in various outfits and shopping apps. All of her social media accounts were secured against hackers, but her photos and text messages would be fair game.

"I can assure you there is nothing in my phone that would help in this investigation," she said flatly.

"So, that's a no?"

Sydney sighed. "No, it's a yes." She leaned back in her chair and folded her arms across her chest. "I have nothing to hide."

"Great," he said, slapping the folder in front of him shut. "It will take some time. I would like to put you up in a local hotel while we continue our investigation."

"But, I need to—"

He raised a hand to cut her off. "We will book you a new

flight to Jamaica. You'll be on your way early tomorrow morning."

Sydney sighed heavily. "Okay."

"In the meantime, there is someone I would like you to meet."

O'Connell nodded at what Sydney assumed was a two-way mirror behind him. Whoever she was about to meet had just heard their entire conversation.

Whether that was a good thing or a bad thing, she was about to find out.

FIVE

SYDNEY

AS THE MINUTES PASSED, Sydney fingered the now cold coffee cup in front of her. She felt more tired than she had since she finished her last half-marathon race. Her eyes felt swollen and puffy, and she was dreaming of a hot shower. A hundred different thoughts were barreling through her mind like a runaway freight train.

She had no concept of time, but it felt as though she'd been waiting inside the small room for hours. O'Connell sat across from her, rifling through his folder of paperwork only peaking up every few minutes in her direction. The room had a faint smell of commercial-grade cleaner, which made her slightly nauseated. Or maybe it was the cocktail of sleeping pills and wine that was still making its way through her system. Just as she was about to ask for a restroom break, the door cracked open.

A broad-shouldered young man with closely cropped brown hair stepped into view. His eyes were a light color that leaned neither to blue nor green; they were a steel grey. He had a straight nose that pointed and a full bottom lip that made him look like a younger Brad Pitt. He was dressed terribly according to Sydney's standards. He wore khaki pants with a brown belt and a pale short-sleeve button-down shirt that was topped off with an equally unfashionable tie.

His fashion choices clearly didn't affect his confidence, because he swaggered his way over to where she was sitting and enveloped her in a faint smell of Old Spice. Sydney fumbled with the long ponytail from her hair extensions and straightened her shoulders.

"This is FBI agent Alex Birch. He will escort you to your hotel," O'Connell said.

He made eye contact with Sydney, and she felted like a wilted flower being burned by the sun.

FBI? This must be serious. She felt a new wave of emotions, mainly panic.

"Mrs. Evans, nice to meet you," said Alex. He moved toward her and extended a large hand to greet her.

She shook his hand weakly and tried to turn up the corners of her mouth. "You too," she said awkwardly as she grasped his hand.

He dropped his hand down to his side and cocked his head. "Please follow me."

She managed to twist her aching body into a standing position, wincing as the sound of the chair scraped loudly across the floor. Dutifully, she followed him out the door. She looked back over her shoulder and saw that Inspector O'Connell was watching them as they walked out. Sydney had a feeling gnawing at her, almost as if they were setting her up for something.

Alex walked silently in front of her, his broad shoulders looming ahead, as they walked down the hall. They stopped at a large black door, which he opened to reveal a room that was much larger than the one she had been questioned in. When she stepped inside, Alex told her to wait by the door.

Folding tables were arranged in long rows with suitcases, carry-on bags, and purses littered across each surface. There was an army of uniformed personnel wearing white latex gloves combing through each bag. She could hear him speaking in a hushed tone to the man who was obviously in charge of the room. The man walked away and returned carrying her vintage purse.

Alex walked back to her and handed it to her. "Need this?"

"Yes, thank you!" she said. Immediately she buried her hand inside as they returned to the hallway. Although there was no phone, Sydney was able to retrieve a pack of mint-flavored gum and stuck a few pieces in her mouth. Between the black coffee and whatever she had eaten on the plane, her breath needed a refresh.

Sydney followed Alex back down the hallway.

"We've set you up in a local hotel for the night. One of the officers will bring your suitcase in a few hours," he called over his shoulder. Sydney was relieved; she always packed a set of fresh clothes and toiletries in her carry-on. At least she would be able to get a shower and put herself back together once she arrived at the hotel.

"What about my cell phone?" she asked.

"It will take a few hours for them to analyze your phone. As I'm sure O'Connell told you, they'll be reading text messages, email, anything related to the investigation." Sydney cringed at the thought of her entire personal life being sifted through by complete strangers. But who was she kidding? Since Jack died, she hadn't had much of a personal life anyway.

"Officer Birch?"

"You can call me Alex," he said, giving her a sideways smile.

"Okay, Alex, is this normal? I mean, to keep someone overnight in a hotel in order to search their phone? It feels... like I am missing something?"

Alex turned his head back slightly to look at her and raised his eyebrows. She couldn't tell if he was surprised or impressed. He shrugged.

"Your case is a little different, Mrs. Evans."

Different how? she wondered. She wanted to press him for more information but decided to wait until she had a chance to think through things more.

"Okay." She looked down at her purse limply banging against her leg as they walked down the hall. She looked at him again. "You can call me Sydney."

As he pulled open the large glass door leading outside, he gave her a half smile that revealed two dimples on each cheek. Sydney tried to smile back, but her throbbing head made it difficult to manage. "We're almost there."

As they stepped into the parking garage, the gravity of the situation began to weigh on her. Rows of neatly parked cars spanned out on either side of her. She walked slightly behind Alex looking at the pavement, as if she were being escorted to the principal's office.

She thought of Marissa and Ethan and wondered if they were in a similar situation to hers. It was a creepy feeling, each of them being questioned in the murder of their friend. *They're innocent,* she kept telling herself. *Try not to worry.* But she was worried. Mainly because her memories of what messages were on her cell phone were a bit foggy at the moment. Were there any messages that could be read the wrong way? That would make Marissa look bad? She didn't communicate with Ethan. After Jack died, they barely spoke to each other. It wasn't that they didn't care about each other, but it was a silent agreement that speaking of Jack or anything else was too painful still.

And poor Lizzy. How could this happen?

She thought back to the day the three of them had met at Northwestern University. It was their sophomore year. Sydney and Lizzy had met in their Advanced Digital Marketing class. They were working together on a project in the library and decided to break for a coffee run. It was late afternoon, and the campus glimmered with a wet sheen of rain left over from another spring storm.

They were walking down an isolated path when they spotted a tall brunette up ahead. Marissa instantly stood out with her completely coordinated outfit and flawless long brown hair.

"I think that's Marissa Schumacher, the heiress," Lizzy whispered in her ear. Sydney had heard she was attending their school, but this the first time she'd seen her on campus.

Just as they were getting ready to turn off the path, she caught a glint of something in the bushes. Sydney slowed for a moment and realized it was a camera. Someone was trying to take pictures of Marissa, which was completely against school rules.

Without thinking, Sydney shouted at the man: "Hey! Heyyy!" She then ran in his direction.

With a loud thump, the man tumbled forward out of the bushes and onto the wet path. His camera equipment spilled out, and she heard a loud crack as a lens must have snapped. Marissa jumped to the side, her eyes searching wildly for the source of all the noise. The man scrambled his equipment together, ran back toward the bushes, and disappeared.

Sydney and Lizzy caught up to Marissa, both out of breath.

"Are you guys all right?" Marissa said, lines of concern crinkling her perfect face.

"That man, he was trying to take pictures of you or something!" Lizzy burst out.

Marissa sighed. "Oh yes, it happens." She looked wearily toward the photographer's escape path, sighed, and then tossed a lock of long auburn hair before looking back at them. "You both are so sweet to come to my rescue. Please, can I buy you coffee or something?"

"Actually we were just heading to Java House. Want to join us?"

Marissa smiled. "Yes, and it's my treat!"

The three of them walked together and laughed about the whole weird situation. After that they were inseparable for the rest of their college tenure.

Thinking of those times brought tears back to Marissa eyes. Crying, however, wasn't doing anyone any good. She had cried enough for the last six months. She felt something switch inside of her, a resolve to bring justice for her sweet friend.

The loud click of a car door opening snapped her back to the present. Alex was holding the door open to a small Ford Focus, and by the freshly vacuumed look of the interior, she assumed it was a rental car. She nodded a thank-you at him as she plopped down in the front passenger seat. It was all she could do to not push the seat back, close her eyes, and pass out then and there.

"O'Connell put you up at the Marriott by the airport. It's nothing fancy, but you won't be there long."

"Sounds great, thanks," she mumbled. After a few turns they were out of the airport parking lot. Looking out the window, she could see long, flat buildings blurring past as they made their way to the hotel. Grey skies hung overhead, and the air was bloated with the impending rainstorm. She wondered again about the events that had transpired while she was blacked out.

"So, how did I get off the plane?" she asked, breaking the silence that hung in the small car.

Alex chuckled. "You don't remember?"

"Um, no?" she said quietly. *This can't be a good sign*, she thought.

"Well..." Alex then relayed a horrific story of how Sydney had completely passed out on the plane ride—to the point where several stewardesses had been called to her chair when her fellow passengers had wondered if she was breathing. They had propped her up and made sure she was buckled in when the plane landed.

When they arrived at the terminal, she woke up briefly, with just enough time to turn to the newlywed couple next to her and throw up all over their laps. The flight attendants stepped in at that point, removed her neck pillow, and hoisted her off the plane.

"At that point," Alex continued, "you were carried out and laid across a few chairs until several airport security officers came, picked you up in their golf cart, and brought you to our office."

Sydney's cheeks burned, and she felt her stomach knot. She pictured her limp body laid across the golf cart as she was paraded toward Security. She said a silent prayer to herself, *Good Lord I hope no one took of picture of that.* She held her meticulously manicured hand over her mouth in horror.

"Oh my gosh, I am so embarrassed," she said, refusing to

look anywhere but out the window as her cheeks continued to burn. "You must think I'm a mess!"

Alex laughed. "Actually, *that* happens *a lot*. You would be surprised. Ambien has become a regular problem at the airport."

They stayed silent the rest of the ride, Sydney too embarrassed to speak of anything else and too exhausted to keep up any type of small talk. She kept her eyes firmly on the world blurring past her, wishing she could find a way to mentally escape. She felt herself looking around her lap again for her phone. In these situations, it was where she turned to when she needed to lose herself. Therapeutic scrolling through her social media feeds often took her away from the painful realities of her life.

They finally arrived at the hotel, and she nearly leapt out of the car when the bellman opened the door. She felt like a mess and wished she'd packed a baseball cap to hide her matted hair. The sunglasses she pulled from her purse would have to do for now.

After an awkward check-in at the hotel desk (where the clerk thought they were a couple), Alex escorted her to her room. As they walked down the hall, two police officers turned the corner toward them. Sydney eyed them cautiously.

"Are those guys for me?" she asked Alex.

"Sorry, it's standard procedure. Just until morning—we need to make sure you don't flee."

Sydney almost laughed. "I'm not the fugitive type."

Alex stopped and looked at her, as if he was sizing her up. "People do strange things when they are under stress," he said as he opened her door.

She wondered how he would define strange. This entire situation felt incredibly strange to her. "I'll let you know as soon as I hear anything, Sydney. Until then, try to get some rest."

"Thanks," she said as she entered the room.

Sydney turned the deadbolt on the door and heaved a sigh of relief. All the embarrassment and fear she'd been holding in since she woke could finally escape from her. She leaned back against the door, sank to the floor, and began to cry.

After a few moments of self-indulgent pity, she reminded herself again that crying wasn't going to help anyone and it certainly wouldn't help find Lizzy's killer. She wiped her face, which was nearly makeup-free at this point, stood up, and headed toward the bathroom. The room was simple: a queen-size bed sat in the center facing a large dresser with a flat-screen TV sitting on top and a small desk and chair in the corner.

As she passed the large beveled mirror to the right of the TV, she got the first glimpse of herself. Smeared makeup. Hair matted on one side. She looked gaunt and pale despite her spray tan.

What a sight the good folks at Homeland Security got to enjoy, she thought as she wiped a tear from her cheek.

Her shirt was wrinkled, and her jeans were stained with some type of liquid. It was a far cry from the perfectly poised @SydneyStyle11 profile her followers on Instagram saw. Sydney's brand was easygoing, casual chic. She was meant to look effortless but behind the scenes was heavy with preparation. Her transformation had happened over time, one beauty experiment at a time. First she had lost ten pounds, then she went from brunette to blond. She had started wearing false eyelashes, and hair extensions came soon after. Weekly manicures, pedicures, and spray tans kept her looking as polished as a fresh-out-of-the-box

Barbie doll. Her dad, who was always supportive of anything Sydney had done, had even commented, saying, "Is my daughter still in there?" It had taken her years to create that look that all her followers admired.

Where she excelled as an influencer was finding locations that made her outfits pop. A pink-and-white striped top was the perfect contrast to a bright blue brick wall. Palm trees of whatever fabulous beach vacation she was on would complement her straw fedora and gauzy caftan dress.

It began as a hobby. She was working as an account manager at an advertising firm in downtown Chicago. Catering to high-maintenance clients who never seemed happy was a soul-sucking job for Sydney. But she handled it with style, right down to her Tory Burch wedges. Each night she would come home, edit, and post her outfit for the day.

She followed a few other girls who were doing the same thing. A few of them had even quit their full-time jobs to pursue careers as influencers, basically just people who market products to their social media audience. Just a few months into posting herself, she received a flood of messages from fans asking where she bought her clothes and how she did her hair. At that point, she realized she was onto something.

As her following grew, so did her obsession with perfection. The perfect messy bun to match her athleisure look. Every vacation, every trip to the local grocery store had a carefully selected outfit that fit her brand. And although her outfits looked casually chic, behind the camera was a massive spreadsheet of shirts, leggings, dresses, and shoes with hyperlinks to grow her affiliate empire. When she discovered that you could make good money by building the perfect outfit, she was hooked, and influencing became a full-time career.

It was just a few years into this endeavor that she started dating Jack. He was always a happy photographer for her but would never step in front of the camera himself. "That's your thing," he would say. He seemed to adore her neurotic obsession with the perfect shot and always supported her career in fashion blogging. It was only in the last few months before his death that he seemed more annoyed at having to stop at every meal and take a picture. They stopped traveling together as much, and he seemed to pull away from her.

Sydney couldn't think about that right now. Jack was gone and now Lizzy—there was nothing she could do to change the facts. What she really wanted was to sink into the sheets with her phone and scroll through the next two hours of her feed. Alas, there was no phone. So she settled for a hot shower and a warm towel. She still had the towel wrapped around her head as she melted into the freshly made bed sheets and immediately fell asleep.

SIX
SYDNEY

SYDNEY FELT the rumbling begin again, but when she awoke she was on a different plane. Smaller. A five-point harness held her tightly against a small bucket seat. A cockpit curved around her head. Buttons and gauges dotted the convex shape, flashing red and green lights like a Christmas tree. A large bubbled window stretched out before her.

As she looked to her left, she saw him. Jack. *What was Jack doing here?* she thought. Sydney opened her mouth to speak to him, but no words came out. She tried again, but her voice was gone. Sydney's heart began to race. *Jack!* She tried to say the words: *You have to turn back, you can't go, it's too dangerous.*

Jack wouldn't look at her. He was wearing the black headset she had bought him for his birthday. He looked relaxed and in control. The plane dipped wildly, sending her hair floating in the cockpit around her like a halo. Again Sydney tried to scream, tried to tell him what was coming. The sun slid into the frame of the cockpit window, and the glare blinded both of them. Its piercing light grew bright and brighter until everything was white.

SYDNEY BOLTED UPRIGHT. She was still in her bathrobe, white bath towel wrapped loosely around her head. She was drenched in sweat. Another nightmare. *When will they stop?* She touched her stomach and felt a pang of hunger mixed with nausea.

Sydney looked around the room and got her bearings. The television sitting atop the carved wood cabinet was still stuck on the hotel menu screen. She could see her purse in the corner atop her stacked clothes from yesterday's flight. As she brushed her hair from her face, she remembered why she was there. *Poor Lizzy.*

Sydney stumbled from the bed and spotted a tiny coffee maker on a small shelf near the bathroom. She dragged her feet in that direction. As the coffee popped and gurgled, she heard a brisk knock at the door. She peered out the peep-hole and saw the bellman standing patiently with her suit-case. *Finally!* She nearly shrieked with pleasure.

Sydney needed her armor of makeup, clothes, and accessories to face what was next, whatever that might be. As far as she knew, Lizzy's killer was still at large. She was determined to take the heat off Marissa and Ethan and help the police find the true criminal.

She pulled the suitcase inside, tossed it on the bed, and unzipped the inside compartments. Her neatly packed suit-case was now a bit disorganized and the contents a tad crumpled, but Sydney was so elated to have a little bit of her life back she didn't care. The next hour was spent making up the social media image that most of her friends knew her for—chic, put together, and entirely in control.

She quickly applied her signature "Five-Minute Makeup Routine." In truth, it took fifteen minutes (or more) to create her daily look, but her fans loved it anyway. She pulled on a pair of artfully torn jeans, a fresh white T-shirt, and a buttery-soft long cashmere sweater that dusted her calves. Delicate gold hoops and leather ballet flats finished her look. It felt a little hollow, worrying about what she looked like when she had just lost her friend. But experience told her otherwise. When you felt put together on the outside, it made facing the crazy world a little bit easier to handle.

As she worked her curling wand through her hair, she thought about Lizzy. How could someone so sweet have any enemies, much less someone who would want to take her life? Will seemed too clean-cut to do anything so foul as murder. But he was there, probably drinking alongside her. Maybe he could tell Sydney something about the plane ride that he hadn't told the authorities. She made a mental note to seek him out as soon as they arrived at the resort.

The inspector had also mentioned Lizzy's work at the offices of DoubleDownCasino.com. She knew Lizzy hadn't worked there long, and she had told her several times that the job had been a lifesaver for her financially. But Sydney also remembered her complaining about Alice, Ethan's secretary. Alice was an older woman in her midfifties. She was pencil thin, with stick-straight red hair that she parted down the center and always kept in a tight bun. Sydney had met her several times while visiting Jack, and she'd always given her an uneasy feeling, like she was hiding something. *Maybe Lizzy found out her secret.*

Any further ruminations were halted by a sharp knock at the door. Alex was waiting on the other side. He didn't know it, but she was about to prove to him that Marissa and Ethan were innocent.

SEVEN

MARISSA

THE SOFT BUT firm knocking was insistent. Marissa thought she was dreaming, but as she pulled the silk embroidered sleep mask away from her eyes and peered across the softly lit room, she realized it was coming from the door. At first, she looked around the carefully decorated honeymoon suite with a sense of peace. It was everything she had dreamed of when they booked El Brillo Azul for their wedding. The morning light was just barely creeping through the slits in the large heavy aquamarine-colored curtains on the far side of the room.

As she sat up in bed, it hit her: *Lizzy is gone.* She tapped a finger to the bags under her eyes, still swollen from her tears the night before, as if to confirm it was real. A dull ache had formed behind her forehead, a remnant of the shock and stress she had endured the day before. She sat up and looked over at Ethan, who was still sleeping soundly next to her. One taunt, muscular arm was tossed lazily over the right side of his face, hiding the angular cut of his jaw.

Their arrival in Jamaica was met with a fanfare of flashing red lights. Fire trucks, ambulances, and several police vehicles swarmed the tarmac ahead of the jet wheels touching the ground. The paramedics entered the plane and confirmed what they all knew to be true: Lizzy was indeed dead. Though a medical examiner would need to confirm the cause of death, it looked as though she had suffered from cardiac arrest.

Ethan took the news with a stoic nod while Will just stood there with a wild look of shock in his eyes. Marissa nearly passed out—Ethan had to practically carry her inside the airport while they removed the body from the plane. As she sat inside the gated waiting area and stared out the large window, the medics worked frantically to take her vitals.

She felt fine; whatever had stopped Lizzy's heart was limited to only her. Once the three of them had been checked out and cleared for any signs of illness, the interrogations began. It was clear to her by the way the police handled the situation that they believed Lizzy's death was not from natural causes.

Will, Ethan, and Marissa were separated into three different rooms, and they each spent hours answering question after question about what happened on the plane. Marissa was so shocked and frankly sad that she barely remembered what she told them. The whole experience was a blur.

There was one particular question, however, that stood out in her mind.

"Miss Shumacher, do you have any reason to believe your husband would want to hurt Miss Ortez?" the dark-skinned investigator asked her with a thick Jamaican lilt. The question had completely caught her off guard; the thought had not occurred to her at all. She knew Lizzy was working in Ethan's office, but that was the only contact or relationship they had ever had.

"Ethan? Of course not. Lizzy is a dear friend of ours. We loved her." She stared off to the corner of the room, as the words caught in her throat.

"Of course, of course," he said and looked back down at the yellow note pad in front of him. She returned her gaze from the corner of the room and noticed he was making notes. She couldn't read his writing, but the whole exchange gave her an uneasy feeling.

When the sun dipped below the crystal blue ocean, she was finally released. A black town car was waiting to take her and Ethan to the resort. Even though Will was nowhere in sight, Marissa was too exhausted to worry about him. She slumped into the black leather seat and fell asleep on Ethan's shoulder.

So that morning, as she rose to answer the door, was the first time since she left the airport that she had even had a chance to think about what to do next. And a tiny voice in the back of her mind warned her that things might not be as they seemed.

She shook away any more dark thoughts, wrapped herself in a pale pink silk robe, and pulled open the door.

"Sorry to interrupt you, madam, but you have a meeting this morning with the event planner in thirty minutes," said Simon, the personal butler who had been assigned to them for their stay.

Simon was a willowy figure, who looked to be in his late sixties. He had probably been as tall as Ethan when he was young, but the years had given him a slight bend in his back. He stooped over a silver tray of steaming coffee and pastries and gave her a timid smile. "And I've brought you some coffee."

"No, it's fine." She mustered up a weak smile and took the tray from his bony hands. "Thank you, Simon."

Ethan was awake and stared groggily at her as she sat back down in bed. She placed the silver tray in the swirled sheets next to his long body. She could feel the heat from him as she settled in closer; he had always been a hot sleeper. Part of her just wanted to curl up in his arms and go back to sleep. Instead, she handed him his coffee and crossed her legs.

"I can't believe she's gone. How could someone so young and healthy die from cardiac arrest?" she said. There must have a been a thousand other questions that were rattling through her head at the moment. But it was the first thought that whizzed into her head.

"I don't know." Ethan stared at his coffee after taking a sip. The steam wafted up and shimmered in the morning sunlight. "But the medical examiner and police are investigating her death. So we don't have to worry. I'm sure they will find out what happened."

He placed a hand on her back, gently rubbing the space between her shoulder blades. He knew that was her soft spot. But Marissa didn't care for his answer. He seemed so quick to dismiss the problem and embrace the idea that the police would just handle it. She stared down at her robe and thought again about what the inspector had asked her.

"I'm not so sure. I mean, how great can the Jamaican police be?" She felt like a snob for even thinking it, but she was guessing the Jamaican police force was not exactly a well-funded operation.

"Lizzy's an American citizen. I'm sure they'll send someone from the States to help with the investigation."

Investigation, she thought. It sounded so final, so real. She felt her eyes burn with tears. Ethan seemed to pick up on her distress. He put down his cup and placed his arms around her.

"Listen, there is nothing we can do about it now, honey. We've given our statements. We've cooperated with the police. Let them do their jobs, and we can focus on what's next." He took a deep breath. "Do you still want to go through with the wedding?"

The tears began to flow at that point. Marissa's brain flashed memories of the last few months and all the work Lizzy had done to help her with the wedding. Her friend was genuinely happy for her. Lizzy recognized this was a chance for both her, an orphan, and Ethan, who had lost his twin brother, to start a new life together. She knew her friend wanted that for her. She just didn't know if she had the strength to do it without her.

After what seemed like an eternity, she felt her breathing slow. She began to take some deep breaths, a technique she learned through years of yoga practice. This wasn't just about her; it was a fresh start for all of them. She knew Lizzy would have wanted this for her.

She looked at Ethan sitting next to her, his eyes conveying sympathy and support. She brushed a lock of hair from his forehead.

"Yes, I think we should. For us. And for Lizzy." She took a long drink from her coffee cup as if washing away any last doubts she had about the wedding. "I think that's what she would have wanted."

EIGHT

SYDNEY

WHEN ALEX STEPPED into her room, Sydney immediately noticed his smell. He must have been wearing cologne, a spicy musk that smelled expensive. He had swapped his terrible khaki pants for a thin grey hoodie, skinny jeans, and Nike sneakers. It was a noted improvement that caught her off guard. Sydney was even more surprised when he pulled his hands up and revealed he had brought her breakfast.

"Morning, Sydney. I brought you a cappuccino and pastries," Alex said with a forced smile, thrusting a coffee and paper bag toward her.

"Good morning," she said and quickly grabbed the coffee and brown bag from his hands. "And thank you. I'm starving." Her stomach grumbled at the sight of the food, and she realized it'd been over twenty-four hours since she had eaten anything.

"Unfortunately, you'll have to eat in the car. They want to see you back at the airport, go over the next steps. And"— he gave her an unexpected smile—"you'll get your phone back."

"Thank goodness. I need to talk to Marissa; she must be freaking out right now."

A concerned look fluttered across Alex's face and then quickly disappeared. He bent down and pulled the handle from her suitcase.

"Here, let me grab your suitcase."

"Sure. Thanks."

At least he's being a gentleman, she thought. Having an FBI escort was new territory for her; she wasn't sure what to expect.

As they rode back to the airport, Sydney scarfed down two pastries and practically chugged her cappuccino. She pelted Alex with questions about the investigation, which got her nowhere. He was a citadel of information, impenetrable. She quickly decided she was going to have to change tactics if she was to get any information out of him.

"So, have you ever had to shoot a gun at someone?"

"Yes, once," he said. "But I can't tell you any more." He paused. "It's classified."

"Oh please. I'm sure it's nothing I haven't seen on *Criminal Minds*."

"You watch *Criminal Minds*? That's a bit dark for your taste, isn't it?"

"What is that supposed to mean?" She felt immediately defensive, like he wasn't taking her seriously. But she knew what he was alluding to. It wasn't the first time she'd been underestimated because of her looks, or rather, all the time she spent on her looks.

"I happen to like crime shows. Besides"—she gave him a sideways glance—"I have insomnia, and that show is always on TV."

Alex shrugged, keeping his hands at ten and two on the wheel. It was the first time she noticed the indent on his left ring finger. She'd been on the single scene for long enough to know what that meant. He was either married or recently divorced. He seemed to catch her eyes lingering on his hand and dropped it down on his lap.

"Well, not everything is like you see on TV. I wish we solved every case in just under an hour with a neat little ending and a moral takeaway. But in my work, it's usually much more complicated...and messy."

She sensed he was letting his guard down, and she wondered if he was trying to build trust.

"Like my situation?"

He tipped his chin in her direction as if he was deciding whether to say something more. Instead he just replied with "Yes, you could say that."

The engine rumbled along, keeping a silent hum in the car that buffered the silence between them. Her eyes drifted out the window, and she thought about why she was there. *Lizzy.* The loss was still fresh, but having a full night of sleep at the very least let her regain her facilities.

And at this point, she needed control. Because she felt as if her life was spiraling out of her hands. It was hard to believe she had lost her husband and now one of her closest friends within six months. It didn't seem fair. She blinked rapidly as the tears started to make their way back to her eyes. When Jack disappeared, she wasn't ready to accept he was dead. There was no body, just a few of his personal items. She hadn't accepted his demise until she had proof.

And now, with Lizzy, she wasn't about to let her murder go unsolved. She would do whatever it took to track down Lizzy's killer.

"We're here." Alex's voice cut through her thoughts. He pulled the door open for her and grabbed her suitcase from the trunk. She logged a few steps behind him as they approached the double metal doors leading into the building. With so many thoughts swirling around in her mind, she preferred to skip the small talk.

As they walked down the hallway, Sydney began to feel anxious again. She knew that O'Connell would be waiting with the results of her phone search, and he might have even more news about Lizzy's death. As Alex pulled open the door of the room that she had spent much of her afternoon in yesterday, she took a deep, calming breath and stepped inside.

Her sense of calm was quickly shattered as she sat down across from the giant form of Inspector O'Connell to her left. Alex settled in on her right. Most men would been dwarfed by O'Connell's large frame, but Alex held his shoulders back and straight, making the inspector look like a giant blob. An intense blob, nonetheless.

"Mrs. Evans, thank you for your patience as we sort out this investigation," O'Connell said. His voice sounded garbled, and he spoke as if he hadn't slept. His black hair was damp and glistened in the windowless room. He smelled like a combination of cheap aftershave and burnt coffee. "I'm happy to report that we didn't find anything that would...incriminate you on your phone."

Sydney sat back, surprised at the word he used...*incriminate*?

"Okay, well, that's a good thing, right?"

"It is." His voice was heavy and slow. "So now we need to discuss what's next. Your phone was very helpful to our investigation."

"Helpful? Helpful how?" she said, suddenly feeling off balance. She turned to Alex, but he wouldn't make eye contact.

"The details are not important right now," he said. The

look he was giving her suggested she ought not to pry further. But Sydney was not about to let him off that easy.

"I think I have a right to know what you found on my phone," she snapped.

"You don't have any rights to the knowledge we collect during our investigation, Mrs. Evans, unless we wish to share it with you. This is a delicate situation, as you may have guessed, because Miss Ortez was killed over international waters and now her body lies in a foreign country. So we will do our job the way we see fit, and you will receive pertinent information on a need-to-know basis."

She leaned forward to speak, her frustration at being kept in the dark turning into anger. But just as she was about to open her mouth, she saw Alex shift in his chair. It was subtle, but the small movement made her rethink her strategy.

"Okay, fine. Well, I hope that anything you found on my phone made it clear that Marissa and Ethan had absolutely nothing to do with Lizzy's murder."

"Not exactly." He cleared his throat, an awful, throaty sound that made Sydney blanch. "At this point, we are still pursuing all options in the case. I know you think your friends are innocent, Mrs. Evans." He raised his eyebrows at her, scrunching up the folds of skin hanging on his fore-head. "And I hope you are right. But there are still a lot of questions we need answers to."

Sydney carefully considered what he saying, trying to read between the lines. The room was heavy with all the thoughts and words she knew weren't being said.

"Well, I'm here," she said. "What questions can I answer for you?"

He leaned back again, peering intently at her.

She felt like she was fumbling around in the dark, trying

to listen to words in a different language and understand what it all meant. *Why couldn't he just get to the point?* She felt like there was something he wanted to ask her.

O'Connell finally relented and began to speak. "The best way for us to get the answers we need is to get closer to everyone who was on the plane at the time of Miss Ortez's death. We feel confident that whoever poisoned her had access to the plane. And that narrows down our list of suspects, but...it doesn't give us any leads as to why someone would want her dead." He laid his thick hands flat on the table as he continued on. "We need to get close to Marissa and Ethan, as well as their guests, and see how they behave over the next few days. Mrs. Evans, we need to be at that wedding."

Sydney was floored. "So, you want *me* to spy on my friends?"

"Not exactly. I want you to attend the wedding as planned." He took a deep breath and ran his hands across the top of his glistening head of hair. "The only difference is Officer Birch will be accompanying you as your date."

NINE

MARISSA

JESSICA GAINES, Ethan and Marissa's event planner for the wedding, was standing at attention in the lobby looking as though she'd already downed five espressos. There was a quiet morning hum around the space as servers and butlers crossed the marble-tile floors, carrying trays with food domes and coffee. Marissa could smell bacon cooking off in the distance along with the sweet aroma of fresh baked goods. The smells would have comforted her, but today they felt bittersweet.

"Good morning, darlings," Jessica said with a sympathetic smile as they arrived in the elegantly appointed lobby. She wore thick red glasses and had a sharply cut black bob that made her look a little like a cartoon character. She was always dressed in a freshly pressed black suit with utilitarian black flats that only accentuated her short stature. She wore very few pieces of jewelry; however, Jessica always had an expensive Louis Vuitton or Gucci purse in her hand, as if to signify her success.

Marissa and Ethan had to lean down to greet her as they exchanged a quick hug.

"Sorry we are late, Jessica. We needed to talk this morning...after what happened," Marissa said, giving a sideways glance to Ethan. He nodded silently, letting her take the lead.

"Oh, I know, I know. I heard about what happened." Jessica looked down at her hands, as if to convey her sorrow. "Elizabeth was a sweet, kind girl." She reached for Marissa's hand and patted it gently. Marissa had to push back tears. She appreciated the gesture, even if it felt a little forced.

While she was dressing for their meeting, she wondered how the world-renowned event planner would handle the whole situation. Jessica did not hide her ambition. She had a long list of celebrity weddings under her belt, many of which were featured in *Us Weekly*, *Vanity Fair* and even *Vogue*. Marissa had agreed to let their nuptials be documented in exchange for a big cut in Jessica's fees. She had not wasted any time flying down photographers and journalists to cover the event.

Marissa would bet money that Jessica had never let a wedding falter under her eager yet steady hand. But she doubted murder of a bridesmaid had ever been on the table.

"I've asked Simon to have your breakfast ready at the pergola overlooking the beach so you eat comfortably while we talk," Jessica said, extending a black-clad arm toward the area.

Marissa could see a private table and chairs set up along the beach, with a full spread of food waiting for them. She kept close to Ethan as they left the shelter of the resort lobby and walked toward the beach. He kept a hand around her waist as they walked, the warmth from his body giving her a small bit of comfort. She could feel Jessica's eyes on them as she trailed silently in their wake.

Once they had settled into their pale blue upholstered

chairs, Marissa reached for a cup of coffee and gulped it down. The pergola they were under was swathed in white gauze curtains that rose and fell with the wind from the ocean. The day was clear; intense blue skies hung overhead and the sun continued to rise up from the ocean. She could feel the coral maxi dress she'd hastily dressed in become slightly damp and cling to her skin.

Jessica politely waited for them to enjoy a few bites of food in silence before she began to speak. She looked ready to spring, like a race horse waiting at the gates of the Kentucky Derby. Marissa was impressed with her self-control, having kept silent for this long.

"Darlings," she began, "I know you have been through a horrific, unimaginable experience in the last twenty-four hours. You've lost your friend and you have my deepest condolences." She paused and tucked a chunky black sliver of hair behind her ear. "But you are here now, and I'd like to know how I can help."

Marissa slowly placed her fork back on her plate and dabbed a white linen napkin at the corners of her mouth. She began to speak, but Jessica held up a hand and stopped her.

"Just say the word and I can put the entire wedding on hold until you are ready."

Marissa cleared her throat. "Actually, Jessica, we've decided that we'd like to go through with the wedding." She glanced at Ethan, who nodded his support. "We feel that Lizzy would have wanted us to follow through with our plans. We just want to make sure this is done in a way where we are being respectful of her family and her legacy." The last few words stuck in her throat. She paused for a moment to collect herself before continuing. Ethan reached over and put a hand on her back. "We'd like to prepare a statement for you to send to all of our guests." She fumbled with the napkin in her lap. "And we'd also like to pay a small tribute to her during the ceremony."

Jessica's eyes sparkled in response. Marissa could tell she was brimming with joy at the news. Pulling this wedding off with everything that had happened would be a huge coup for her. The media coverage alone would likely have her booked out for years. But despite Marissa's knowledge of her selfish ambitions, she knew that if anyone could handle the situation with grace, it would be Jessica.

"Of course, of course. I think that's a wonderful idea. Don't you worry dears, I will take care of everything."

With a sudden burst of energy, she reached down into a large canvas bag and pulled out her laptop. She began making notes and typing out the notification to guests. Marissa felt herself relax for a moment, knowing she was in capable hands.

Ethan sat next to them in silence as they hammered out the rest of the details for the wedding. She glanced over at him several times, wondering what had him staring off toward the ocean. She wasn't sure if Lizzy's death had sunk in for either of them, but grief aside, neither of them knew what had caused Lizzy's death.

Or rather, *who*.

Just as she began to get distracted with the notion of Lizzy's murder, a large elegant cake stand arrived with small pieces of cake tucked underneath a large glass dome. The professionally dressed waiter opened up the stand, and the smells of fresh baked cake and vanilla-flavored frosting wafted over to them. Thinking about Lizzy had caused Marissa's appetite to leave her, but Ethan didn't seem to mind. He helped himself to a few slices of wedding cake.

"Before I forget," Jessica said, adjusting her red-rimmed

glasses. "We've had a last-minute RSVP to the guest list. Apparently a well-known businessman in the Caribbean." She had raised her eyebrows as she said this, and Marissa wondered why. Ethan paused and looked up at Jessica, his fork suspended in midair with a piece of red velvet cake wobbling on top. "Does the name Vincente Estavez ring a bell?"

Ethan dropped his fork back on his plate. He reached for a one of the tall skinny glasses of water and took a deep drink.

"Oh yes, he's a business associate of mine," Ethan said, clearing his throat.

She couldn't put her finger on it, but something about the way he said it made her uneasy. She had watched Ethan play enough charity poker to know his tell.

Something was wrong.

TEN

SYDNEY

SYDNEY FELT as if someone had dumped a bucket of cold water over her head, which contrasted sharply to the heat that had risen in her cheeks. The room she was in began to fall away, and all she could focus on was the two men in front of her. One asking the impossible, the other she barely knew.

"You want him"—she wagged a finger at Alex—"to go as my *date*?"

"Yes, he will be undercover and will be joining you for observation only."

Sydney made a huffing noise, which seemed to bounce off the walls in the room. Alex looked as though he wanted to speak but kept his lips still. Sydney threw her hands up and brought them down, causing the gold bangles on her wrists to slap against the table. "Do I even have a choice?"

"Yes, you have a choice. But I strongly suggest that you choose to work with us." He took a breath that rattled down his throat. "I wouldn't want to have to charge you with obstruction of justice."

Sydney placed her hands back in her lap. Despite what

he said, she knew she didn't have a choice. Of course, it made sense—law enforcement wanted to get close to everyone involved and see them with their guard down. Asking someone questions in a room like she was sitting in now was way different than having a few cocktails in you and making casual conversation. The latter setting was a much better way to get someone to let a few details slip. *But with a date?* She looked again over at Alex. *No.*

"Okay, I get it. But even if I said yes—which I haven't yet —it would never work."

"And why is that?" O'Connell arched a thick eyebrow at her as he spoke. "You don't think Alex is believable enough? He's roughly your age, single and good-looking."

Sydney raised an eyebrow.

"Is he single? I saw a small indent on his left ring finger. Looks like a mark from a wedding ring to me."

O'Connell and Alex exchanged looks, clearly surprised at her observation. *They shouldn't be impressed*, she thought. Any single girl worth her salt knows the signs of a married man.

"Listen, if I noticed it," she continued, "other women will too. Besides, he is totally not my type."

O'Connell turned his palms up and made a huffing noise.

Alex turned to him and finally broke his silence. "Sir, do you mind if Mrs. Evans and I speak in private?"

"Fine, but don't be long. We are on a short timeline."

Alex nodded and turned his grey eyes to Sydney. "Come on Sydney, let's get some fresh air."

With that he stood up and gestured for her to follow him. Sydney hesitated, looking at O'Connell and then back at Alex. She stood up to follow him.

They retraced their steps down the long grey hallway,

Sydney staying silent as they walked. She knew Alex would be preparing to change her mind, perhaps even put her at ease with the idea of him as her date. Truthfully, it wasn't just that Alex didn't fit the usual profile of someone she would date; it was more about the idea of a *date.* She wasn't ready to have another man taking her arm or doing anything that Jack would have.

Alex pulled open a large glass door leading out to what looked a like a small courtyard within the airport buildings. There was an open grassy area peppered with picnic tables. She could see a couple of airport employees having coffee at the other end of the courtyard. Alex gestured toward a bench off to their right. They sat down next to each other, and Alex turned his body to face her.

"Sydney," he began, "I know this is a lot to take in."

She sighed. "You think?" she said with a touch of sarcasm.

"The truth is, this isn't just about getting justice for your friend, Miss Ortez—"

"Her name was Lizzy."

"Okay, then this isn't just about getting justice for Lizzy. If we don't know who killed her, that means the killer is still out there. We don't have a motive yet, which means we don't know if Lizzy was their primary—or their only—target. And if they had access to the plane, they are likely going to be at the resort where the wedding is taking place. Which means Marissa and Ethan are in very real trouble. You would not only be helping us, but you would be helping to keep them safe as well."

A 747 practically shook their bench as it passed low over their heads and glided down toward the runway. The sound boomed overhead and Sydney held her hands over her ears to dampen the sound.

She knew Alex was right. If the killer was still out there, and if he or she had another target, no one at the wedding was safe.

"So, do you believe that Marissa and Ethan are innocent? That they had nothing to do with this?"

He watched as the plane landed in the distance before turning his attention back to her.

"I believe if you let me come with you, we can find out for sure."

Sydney looked away, trying to decide what to do. She wasn't keen on spying on her friends, but if they were in danger, how could she possibly say no? She was going to have to swallow the idea of having to bring a date, which would draw an uncomfortable amount of attention to her, and accept that she was going to have to spy on her friends all in one bitter pill. She pushed a long strand of hair behind her ear before turning to face Alex again.

"Okay."

"Okay, as in yes, you will work this us?"

"Yes," she said firmly. "But I believe my friends are innocent, and I intend to prove it."

ELEVEN

SYDNEY

ALEX WALKED Sydney back to the interrogation room where O'Connell was waiting. He was standing in the corner of the room, his large bull-like shoulders hunched over as he typed furiously on his phone. She noticed he was pacing in the small corner and wearing reading glasses that made him look like a bespectacled gargoyle. Alex nodded in his direction, indicating the plan was a go. The three of them sat down to discuss what would happen next.

Alex took the lead and laid out the plan for her to assist in the investigation.

"It's pretty simple, Sydney. I just need you to introduce me to your group of friends and that will give me an opening, to ask a few casual questions that might help the investigation."

"Oh, like what? Where you from? And oh, by the way, did you murder the bridesmaid?"

"Not exactly. Listen, Sydney, I know this is...frustrating, but going about things this way helps us get a clearer picture of why someone would want to have murdered your friend."

Sydney sighed. "No, you're right. I want to help."

"Great," he said, pushing his chair back and standing up. "Well, we've got a plane to catch." He turned to O'Connell, who also stood with some effort. "Sir, I'll be in touch."

"Right," he said, nodding. "And remember what we discussed last night."

Alex gave him a wary look. "Of course."

Sydney looked back and forth between the two of them as they exchanged looks. She was definitely going to ask Alex about that when they sat down on the plane.

Alex strode to the door and opened it for her. Two officers were waiting to escort them, holding her suitcase and another that must have belonged to Alex. Another officer approached them and handed Alex something. He turned to her.

"Looks like they got it back to you in one piece," he said, handing her the phone with its jewel-encrusted case.

"Thanks."

She took it carefully and ran her hand over the front. The screen came to life, and she could see she had a ton of notifications waiting for her, but first she wanted to reach out to Marissa.

Marissa! I'm on my way, my flight was delayed. Are you okay? I heard about Lizzy. Devastating. She finished off the message with a tear emoji.

She held the phone down at her side as they walked, trailing behind Alex and the two uniformed officers. Her phone vibrated in her hand.

Sydney! I'm so, so glad you are okay. I was getting worried. I don't even know how to describe what happened, it was awful. We need to talk when you get here. I'm so glad you're coming. I need you.

Don't worry, Sydney typed as she continued to follow the trio of men. *Nothing could stop me from being there.*

Alex looked over his shoulder a few times to check on her. Although she had accepted Alex as her date, she still felt the plan was flawed from the beginning. He was just not believable as her date. While he was kind of cute—she'd give him that—he was just not anything like the kind of guy her friends would expect her to date. She lived in the fashionable world of online bloggers. Every man behind the scenes was styled to perfection. Not to mention that if a guy had no sense of style whatsoever, he wouldn't understand what she did for a living. And therefore, every time she posed in front of a donut shop holding a pink sprinkled donut over her eye, he would be thoroughly annoyed to take fifty pictures.

She suddenly looked around and realized they weren't in the regular terminal. This area had large glass picture windows that went from floor to ceiling, framing out a large concrete air pad that had several medium-size jets waiting on the tarmac beyond.

As the officers opened up the doors and made a beeline for a sleek-looking jet, Alex turned around and smiled at her.

"Ever ridden on a private jet before?" he asked.

"Just once," she said. He raised his eyebrows as if he was waiting for her to elaborate further, but she kept silent. It wasn't a memory she was prepared to share just yet.

"Well, lucky for you, one of the big guns at the bureau just landed here. He was able to spare the plane for a few hours."

The two boarded the plane and settling into reclining seats across from each other, near the front of the plane. After she had stashed her bag and got a drink from the bottle of water sitting next to her chair, she immediately reached down to pick up her phone. Alex settled into his seat and sat silently, occasionally glancing over causally to look out the window. She knew better—he was keeping tabs on her phone. She desperately wanted to google anything about Lizzy's death but didn't want this to seem suspicious. So she went back into her social media feeds and started responding to her followers. This went on for at least ten minutes, Sydney hunched over her phone scrolling through and commenting on her feed and Alex peeking over her shoulder.

"Can I help you?" she finally said.

"Do you always do that?"

"Do what?" she said innocently, tipping her phone away from him.

"Bury yourself in your phone," he said, pointing at the device. "You know, now would be a good time for us to get to know each other. Since I am your date."

"Okay fine," she said, tucking the phone under her leg. "What would you like to know?"

"Well, I've already read your file, so I have the basics. But tell me, what exactly does an influencer do?"

Sydney gave him a tense half smile. She got this question a lot.

"Well, I have a lot of people who follow me on social media, mainly Instagram. I post pictures daily about my life, mostly of what outfit I am wearing or products I am using. People can click on my photos to buy the merchandise I feature in my post." She fumbled with the edge of her cashmere sweater. Saying this out loud to an FBI agent made it sound a little silly. "I make a commission each time someone buys the products from my photos."

"So, you're like a clothing salesperson?"

"It's called affiliate marketing, actually."

"Right, well that sounds...interesting." The way he

paused before saying *interesting* made her think just the opposite. "You seem to be really good at what you do."

"I am," she said, feeling self-conscious. This was another reason why Alex didn't fit the bill as her date. Someone in law enforcement, whose job affected whether people lived or died, would never understand the significance of what she did. Talking about it with him made her feel insignificant.

Jack, on the other hand, had fit the bill in every way. And at first, Jack was completely supportive of her career. He adored her, so every time she asked him to take her picture, he seemed to truly enjoy it. Her career afforded them a string of fabulous vacations for the short time they were together. Paris, Iceland, Fiji. If there was a beautiful destination that offered a unique backdrop for all her photos, they were there. She meticulously planned each trip, working with corporate sponsors to find the perfect backdrops for their product placements. Whether it was showing off a pair of pink Adidas tennis shoes as she trekked around the cobblestone streets of Paris or fending off the cold weather of Iceland in the latest Columbia parka, she always delivered for her sponsors.

At the beginning of her online career, her focus was more general. She shared photos from her daily life, local restaurants, clothing, and salons. But as her Instagram audience grew, she found that there was a tremendous opportunity to be an affiliate sales representative for a multitude of online clothing retailers. Once she tapped into this line of revenue, her monthly income exploded. Like any good entrepreneur, she doubled down on what was working.

With all that success, however, came a lot of pressure. Sydney felt pressure to look perfect all the time. Not just when she was out socializing or shopping. But even for trips to the grocery store or the dentist, she felt the need to have her style on display. This eventually became a point of contention between her and Jack. He said they could never relax and just enjoy wherever they were—it had to be an opportunity to showcase her fashion work. In fact, he had suggested more than once that she scale back because he could take care of them both financially. That hadn't gone over well with independent-minded Sydney.

She pulled her thoughts back to the present and continued to chat with Alex for the rest of the flight. They had a few things in common: both had grown up in small Midwestern towns, came from semi-normal families, and moved away after college. Just when she was about to ask him about his ex-wife, his phone buzzed.

"Sorry, I've got to take this," he said, ducking into the back of the plane. Sydney peeked over her shoulder to make sure he was out of sight before pulling out her phone from underneath her leg. She popped open the Google app and entered a few phrases. *Elizabeth Ortez dead. Marissa Schumacher dead bridesmaid. Schumacher Evans wedding ruined.* Nothing was coming up.

It was clear to her the news hadn't broken yet. That was a relief. Apparently the authorities were keeping things quiet while they conducted their investigation. She continued searching for any updates from blogs and friends' social feeds, but nothing more came up. A few minutes later when Alex walked back into the room, she reflexively stashed her phone away. She caught the sweet musky scent of his cologne again as he sat down next to her.

"We've got something," he said, roping her in with his steel grey eyes. "A motive."

"A motive? Whose motive?" she said, her heart beating a little faster.

74

"It's Will, her live-in boyfriend. O'Connell ran down his information after you suggested we look into him. It turns out he did have a life insurance policy on Lizzy." He took a deep breath before continuing. "To the tune of one million dollars. He was the sole beneficiary. Which is clear motive. Nice work."

Sydney nearly gasped. She felt shocked, horrified, and slightly validated all at the same time. She really didn't expect her hunch about Will would be right; she was just trying to buy some time for Marissa and Ethan. While she wasn't a huge fan of Will's, it still made her sad to think that someone Lizzy cared about so much might betray her like that. *Poor Lizzy*, she thought.

"Wow," she said, recovering from the news. "I honestly didn't expect that."

"You work cases like this long enough and you will find that people will often surprise you." He looked to the front of the plane as the seatbelt light came back on. "And not in a good way."

Sydney was quiet for a moment, taking in the news.

There was a scurrying of activity as a flight attendant appeared and the pilot announced their imminent arrival.

"Well, at least we know one thing," she said, breaking her silence.

"What's that?" Alex said, looking back at her.

"We know who we need to talk to first."

TWELVE

SYDNEY

AS SYDNEY and Alex stepped out into the tropical Jamaican heat, just outside the airport doors, she felt her shoulders slump and relax. The palm trees swayed lazily in the tropical breeze. The sun bathed the entire landscape in bright warm sunshine. Travelers were bustling around the parking lot ahead of her, joining their friends as they boarded various private transport vans taking them to their respective destinations.

In another time and place, this would have been a welcome change of pace. Now, however, was not the time to let her guard down. Sydney was still trying to process what had happened and what her role in all of this was. For the first time in months, her thoughts weren't focused on her online media presence or her grief. Here friends needed her help, and that suddenly took priority.

She was determined to bring justice for Lizzy, but she was starting to realize, even justice had a cost. If Will was truly responsible for her death, the ripple effects would be devastating. How could someone they knew, someone in their circle of friends, commit such a heinous act against one of their own? How would Lizzy's and Will's families react when they heard the news?

Sydney adjusted the heavy vintage bag on her shoulder, shifting uncomfortably in the sun. She had slipped into the restroom of the airport lounge and changed out of her travel attire and into a white eyelet romper and beige Tory Burch sandals. She finished off her outfit with a multilayered gold necklace and wide-brimmed sun hat. Normally she would have been reaching out to anyone passing by to take a picture of her outfit so she could post it to her account. But as soon as her followers found out about what had happened to Lizzy, posting photos of her outfit would seem insensitive. And they would be right in their judgement. However, her portrayal on social media was what kept her in control. Nothing in her life felt under her control anymore.

Alex suddenly appeared by her side, carrying two Red Stripe beers. Sydney raised an eyebrow as he popped the top off both beers and handed one to her.

"Drinking on the job?" she said.

"It's undercover work," he said with a slightly mischievous smile.

Sydney didn't know quite what to make of this. It was possible that he was trying to break down her defenses so that he could get more intel from her or build trust. Either way, she was so tense in that moment, that a beer was perhaps just what she needed to clear her head. She retrieved the cold glass bottle from his hand and let the cold amber liquid slide down her throat. They walked toward their shuttle, falling in step with each other.

As they approached the shuttle that would take them to Montego Bay, a large man with a wide smile, and an equally wide girth, stepped out. He had on a white polo that clung to his bulging midsection and was carefully tucked into his khaki pants. She could see a printed name tag dangling from his left breast pocked as he approached, but she couldn't quite make out his name. He wiped the sweat from his brow as it beaded up in droplets from the warm sunlight that flooded the parking lot.

"Welcome to Jamaica, my friends! My name is Marcel, and I am your driver today." He reached out and eagerly shook hands with each of them. Sydney had to wipe a little sweat from her palms after they shook hands. "Are you here on your honeymoon?"

"Uh, well…" Sydney began, trying to come up with the right words.

"Nope, we're just dating," Alex jumped in. He threw his arm around Sydney and pulled her into him tightly. Sydney immediately tensed up. "But if all goes well, maybe there's a proposal in the future."

She pushed him away playfully. "If you're lucky," she said, recovering. She could feel her cheeks flush with heat, but she still managed to give Alex a reprimanding look.

As Sydney and Alex climbed inside the van, they discovered another couple would be joining them. Sandy and Dan Silva were middle-aged Canadians who made a yearly pilgrimage down to Jamaica to enjoy the beauty of the island and escape from the cold winters of their home.

Alex made light conversation with the jolly couple. Sydney said a polite hello but then stared out the window and sipped her beer.

With Alex distracted, she pulled out her phone and started searching for everything she could find on Will. She reread a few text messages from Lizzy, but nothing she found revealed any discord between the two of them. Lizzy only spoke of their date nights, the new puppy they had brought home. She pulled up both of their social media feeds, each showing a series a photos of them as a couple. The first few photos she saw of Lizzy's face, with a big bright smile framed out by a halo of black curls, brought the sting of tears to her eyes. She had to take a few deep, calming breaths and a swig of her beer before she could continue.

Alex seemed to notice her change in demeanor and pulled his attention away from his new friends.

"You okay?" he said, his voice heavy with sympathy.

"Yes, I was just—" she caught herself, wondering if she should include him on her ideas about Will. "I was just looking at Lizzy's and Will's social media feeds. Seeing if there was anything that might show a rift between them."

"And what did you see?" he said, peeking over at her phone.

Sydney sighed. "Nothing really. They actually looked happy," she said, the disappointment heavy in her voice. He leaned closer to her and she scrolled down through the photos she had found.

"Well, social media never tells the whole story. I'm sure you know that," he said dismissively.

"What is *that* supposed to mean exactly?" she said, feeling immediately on the defense.

"I just mean that most people only put their best foot forward on their social media. No one likes to air their dirty laundry for everyone to see." He looked at her intently as if he was trying to read her response. "I'm not saying there is anything wrong with only sharing the positive side of your life. It's just most of the time, it's not real."

Sydney made a puffing noise. "Well, sometimes it's real. Some people just have a really great life."

Alex lifted his shoulders and cocked his head. "I'm sure you're right," he said before taking a long drag from his beer.

Sydney rolled her eyes and turned her body away from

him slightly, facing out the window. The rest of the van seemed to have settled down as well as they all fell silent.

Sydney watched as they drove past the rolling hills of Jamaica sprawled out under the hot sun. Through the window on her right, she saw a vast blue ocean and pale sand beaches. The opposite side featured fruit stands, pastel concrete buildings with crumbling paint, and a noticeable amount of barbed-wire fencing. Half the buildings were abandoned, or at least they looked that way until some shirtless Jamaican man appeared through the front doorway.

She started tearing away the damp label on her beer, wondering if Alex was right. She didn't even know what was real in her life anymore. Her husband had died mysteriously in a plane crash, and now one of her dearest friends had been murdered. But if you scrolled through the Instagram feed of @SydneyStyle11 all you would see is one bright sunny day after another with a pearly white smile to match.

She felt lucky to have such a desirable career, but lately, it felt like a drain on her soul. She was so much more than perfect makeup and front-tucked T-shirts with quirky sayings like "no coffee, no talky." Sydney had all the elements perfectly down: the right pose to elongate her legs, the just-so smile with her overdrawn lips. But even though she kept the work up at a frantic pace when Jack died, being an Instagram celebrity lost a little bit of its soul. So much of her life since then felt made up, which is why Alex's comment stung.

The challenge for her now was what would she do otherwise?

Her thoughts were interrupted when she heard a loud boom and felt the van lurch to the right. Sydney grabbed the fabric seat back in front of her and braced herself as the van moved violently from side to side. She could see the driver grip the steering wheel with both hands, frantically trying to steer the vehicle in a straight line. As he pumped the brakes, she felt her body snap forward, causing her safety belt to tighten on her chest. A loud honking noise grew louder behind them, and something in her mind told her to brace for impact.

The screeching sound of metal against metal exploded in her ear drums as a car slammed into the back of their vehicle. The van wobbled precariously for a moment, and she wondered if they might topple over, but eventually the swaying stopped. Sydney had squeezed her eyes shut before the car hit them from behind and slowly opened them to survey the damage.

"Sydney, are you okay?" Alex asked as he unbuckled his seatbelt, facing her.

"I...I think so," she said, her voice trembling.

He reached out to her and grasped her head between her hands, looking into her eyes. Then he ran his hands down her sides, searching for any damage to her body. Sydney could see beyond his shoulder that the Jamaican hills were now on her right side; the van had made a complete one-hundred-and-eighty-degree turn. They were facing the wrong side of the road, and the van had landed in a low ditch.

"Is everyone all right?" Marcel called from the driver's seat. He turned around to face them, a small trickle of blood running down his forehead.

"We're fine," replied Alex, turning away from Sydney to look at the rest of the passengers. Dan Silva had not been so lucky. She saw his body crumpled on the floor and his wife, Sandy, hunched over him, her hands cradling the sides of his face.

"Dan, are you all right?" she said, the panic rising in her voice.

His response was a moan as he rolled over to make eye contact with her. He had a small gash on the side of his head, which seemed to be swelling before their eyes. To Sydney's relief, that seemed to be his only wound. Alex left his sea t and knelt down next to him.

"Can you hear me, Dan?" asked Alex. The man blinked a few times and tried to focus on his wife.

"Yes," he said weakly.

Alex looked at the pupils of his eyes and then up at the driver. "He probably has a concussion. Can you call an ambulance?"

"Yeah mon, no problem." Marcel grabbed his phone and dialed 112 for emergency services. After he had relayed the information to the attendant, he phoned the transport company he worked for. "Help is on the way," he said, gesturing to the man on the floor.

Dan was now in sitting position. He seemed to be collecting himself. "I'm sorry," said Dan to his wife, reaching up to touch his head with a shaking hand. "I shouldn't have taken my seat belt off."

His wife did not respond but simply reached over to hug him.

Sydney was touched by the gesture. Seeing the way she comforted her husband made Sydney feel vulnerable and alone.

"I'm going to see what happened," Marcel called back to them as he unbuckled himself and exited the van.

"Wait here," Alex said, tapping her leg. He pried open the sliding door and followed Marcel.

Sydney, unsure of what to do next, grabbed one of her travel scarves out of her bag and handed it to the couple.

"Here, take this for the bleeding," she said, handing it to Sandy.

"Thank you," said Sandy as she looked up at her with watery eyes.

"I'll be fine," interjected Dan. He sat up and placed her scarf on his head. As Marcel and Alex walked around the van inspecting the damage, Sydney and the Canadian couple sat silently. She was too stunned to say or do anything, even take a picture with her phone. Fifteen minutes of this tense silence went by before the ambulance arrived.

While the paramedics insisted on checking out everyone in the van, only Dan required a visit to the hospital. As they loaded him into the back of the emergency vehicle, she could see Sandy holding his hand the entire way. Sydney was touched by the gesture of support and was again reminded that she was alone, except for Alex, whom she hadn't decided she could fully trust yet.

Alex walked up to Sydney as she made her way back toward the van. He had been pacing up and down the road, talking quietly on the phone. He dropped his phone back into his pocket when he reached her.

"How are you feeling?" he asked. He looked genuinely concerned.

"I'm fine. Just a little shook up," said Sydney as she pulled a hat out of her bag and pushed up her sunglasses. "How long did they say it would take before another car arrives for us?"

"I'm not sure. It could be a while," he said with a shrug.

"So, what caused the crash?"

"Marcel thinks we blew a tire," he said.

"You don't sound too sure of that," she said, fingering her wavy blond hair nervously.

"Well…" he said, dropping his hand into his right pocket, "the tire was blown. But I don't think it was an accident. Come with me," he said, wrapping his arm around her as they walked farther up the road, away from Marcel and the van.

Sydney looked around as they walked. The accident had left them stranded on the side of a gravel-lined road. To their right was a rocky beach with trees hanging over a long drop down to the ocean. To their left the hills rose up then fell inland. She could see a few low buildings up at the top of the hill, but they were far from inviting. It appeared as if they had been stranded out in the middle of nowhere. When they crested a small hill, Alex dropped his arm back to his side and turned to face her.

Sydney began to feel anxious. That feeling escalated when Alex reached into his pocket and pulled out a small silver object. It looked like a mini crumbled soda can.

"Is that a bullet?" Sydney in a loud whisper, the shock registering in her voice.

"Shh. Yes, I found it lying next to the tire after it had deflated."

"So, someone shot out our tire? Why?" she said. Her mind raced with possibilities.

"I don't know yet. But if they were able to shoot out our tire, then they had the option to take us out as well. But they didn't." Alex scanned the countryside around him.

She could hear seagulls squawking in the distance as he spoke.

"It was a warning, Sydney," he said, refocusing his eyes on her. "Someone doesn't want us at the wedding."

"Who…who would do that?" Her voice shook as she spoke. Sydney had to hold back tears, as the new revelation hit her. Here she was in a foreign country, with a man she barely knew, who was hired to escort her to this wedding. It seemed that not only had her friend been murdered, but she was now in danger herself. She took a deep breath and tried to steady herself.

Alex seemed to sense her change in demeanor. He dropped the bullet back into his pocket and placed his hand on her arm.

"I wish I had more answers, but right now, we just need to keep going. I've got an agent who will pick up the bullet once we reach the hotel and run some tests. Once we have the results, we'll know more about where it came from." He raised his other hand and now held her gently with both his hands on her arms. "You're doing great, Sydney. You've been very brave."

"Brave?" she said, adjusting her glasses. "I'm scared out of my mind right now."

As she spoke, she turned to see a white van approaching about twenty yards down the hill. She could see Marcel waving wildly for them to stop. Alex dropped his hands as he saw the van approach.

She looked back at Alex. "But, I've come this far and nothing is going to keep me from going to this wedding."

With that, she turned and began stamping down the hill.

.

THIRTEEN
SYDNEY

SYDNEY AND ALEX'S van pulled inside the circular driveway of an expansive resort. Long white buildings accented with pale blue tiles and arched doorways welcomed them with all the glamour of the Caribbean. As she stepped out of the vehicle, she took in the Spanish-style architecture that combined a clay tile roofline with modern glass windows. Carefully selected rattan furniture with plush white cushions was scattered throughout the front breezeway for guests to stop and have refreshing drinks. Giant potted palms, which were kept swaying by a collection of wooden leaf-shaped ceiling fans, seemed to wave hello. El Brillo Azul in Jamaica offered everything you would expect from stylish luxury.

Sydney took a deep breath as two bellhops quickly appeared and retrieved their luggage from the van. She brushed her long blond hair off her shoulders as they stepped outside. She had stashed her cashmere sweater in her carry-on, and her bare shoulders burned from the heat of the sun. Alex stayed close to her as they stepped inside the resort and approached the front desk. They were intercepted by a tall, thin black man wearing a tuxedo. He had thick creases around his eyes that deepened with his smile.

"Mrs. Evans and Mr. Birch, I presume?"

Sydney and Alex looked cautiously at each other. "Yes," they said simultaneously.

"Welcome to El Brillo Azul." He waved his arm wide as he spoke, gesturing to the lobby. He then bowed slightly in their direction. "My name is Maxwell. I will be your personal butler for the duration of your stay."

Sydney and Alex both nodded and smiled as he spoke.

"We have upgraded you to a honeymoon suite so that you can be more comfortable together." Maxwell smiled as he said this, making the implications quite clear.

"Oh, that won't be necessary," Sydney said, interrupting his accented speech. "We can just stay in a regular room with two beds."

Maxwell frowned at this, as if he didn't understand. "You are not together?" he said, pointing from Sydney to Alex and back again.

She felt Alex wrap his arm around her shoulders.

"Of course we are," Alex said, giving her a little squeeze. "Sydney is just shy. We'd love to see the honeymoon suite. Please, lead the way, Maxwell," he continued, extending his arm forward.

Maxwell smiled again, seemingly satisfied with his answer.

"My pleasure," he said, bowing slightly again. He turned on his heel and began walking down the hallway on their right. Alex kept his arm around Sydney as they took the first few steps, then dropped them when Maxwell began gesturing to various spots around the resort, giving them a verbal tour of the space. Sydney glanced at him, expecting a reprimand, but he kept his eyes forward until they arrived at their room.

Maxwell opened the door to a large open room with a four-poster bed and modern accent furniture. The curtains were pulled back to reveal a sweeping view of the ocean framed by potted palms and a charming bistro set on the balcony. On the bed were rose petals fluttering from the wooden fan churning above. They were laid out in the shape of a heart. Sydney could feel her cheeks burning as they stood awkwardly at the foot of the bed.

"Sydney," Alex began once Maxwell had closed the door behind him, "we need everyone to believe we are dating. Even Maxwell."

Sydney didn't respond. She couldn't pull her eyes away from the flower petals. They were just like the ones that she and Jack had found in their own honeymoon suite, just a year ago.

Jack had surprised her with a last-minute trip to Aruba, a chance for them to break away from work. She had happily agreed to the trip and immediately began planning outfits and images for her social media feeds. Jack had a different idea.

"What if we just escaped everything, your job and mine? No photos, no interruptions, just you and me?" he had said. If it was anyone else she would have said no, but he had a way of sweeping any doubts from her mind.

"Yes," she had said with a kiss.

It wasn't long after their arrival that Jack proposed. He wanted to get married that evening, just the two of them in a small ceremony. The idea of eloping had not been on Sydney's radar, but Jack's enthusiasm was irresistible. At first, it felt crazy—she had always thought of having a big wedding. The photos alone would have gained her another thousand followers on her Instagram account. But there was something about eloping that also felt exotic and special, an intimate affair they alone were privy to.

And so she had agreed. She and Jack had married on a pristine white beach in Aruba, joined only by a small cast of employees from the resort where they were staying. They were deliriously happy, and Jack had carried her over the threshold of their hotel suite then dropped her on a bed covered in flower petals.

Just like the ones she was staring at now. She felt a ball of emotions harden in her stomach.

"Sydney?" Alex said, touching her arm. He startled her out of her thoughts.

"Yes, sorry," she said finally looking his way. "You were saying?"

"I was saying that we need to be more convincing, as a couple." He cocked his head, his grey eyes shimmering from the sunlit beach behind her. "The more people are convinced we are a couple, the more likely they will be to let their guard down. And help us find Lizzy's killer."

"You're right," she said, burying her thoughts of the past. "I'm sorry."

She walked to the credenza under the wall-mounted TV and picked up a piece of gilded stationery that lay underneath. It was a printed itinerary for the weekend informing her that there would be a cocktail hour starting at 6:00 p.m., with light appetizers by the piano bar overlooking the ocean.

"The cocktail hour has already begun. But I know this crowd, I'm sure everyone will still be there for hours." She looked back at Alex, who had walked over to the large glass doors overlooking the beach. "I think we have just enough time to shower. Mind if I go first?"

"Of course. Be my guest," he said not turning around. She wondered what he was looking for as he faced the long stretch of beach. Sydney grabbed a few toiletries from her suitcase and headed to the bathroom on the other end of the room. After a quick shower, she wrapped herself in the fluffy white hotel robe and stepped back into the main room.

"You're up," she said as she stepped out of the bathroom.

"Thanks," he said as he passed her. She noticed Alex had laid out his evening clothes on the bed. Sydney tossed her dress and accessories next to his. Something about their clothes laying side by side on the bed made her sad. It was too familiar, too similar. She wasn't ready for another man in her life yet. She realized her hands were shaking slightly, as her nerves had started to get the best of her. *Maybe a drink would help.* She noticed a fully stocked bar near the door to the room.

She found some cold Diet Coke stocked in the refrigerator, poured it over a fresh cup of ice, and added a shot of rum. *Make that two shots*, she thought, pouring another. A few swigs later and Sydney felt a little more relaxed. It was impossible to process the situation mentally, because the sheer gravity of it threatened to knock her over like a tidal wave. She was anxious to see Marissa but also dreading it.

Sydney was not a good liar.

She was sure that Marissa would pick up on her uneasiness and forced behavior. Not to mention, they needed to talk about Lizzy. Facing Marissa meant facing the truth that her friend was gone. She walked to the other end of the room and pulled open the wide glass door leading out to the balcony. There was a small private hot tub bubbling quietly just outside their door.

The beach stretched out in front of the window.

Thatched roof cabanas shaded soft lounge chairs that were set in pairs to welcome the next couple. The water was dotted with anchored boats quietly waiting to host guests on their next excursion. A couple of young men in life jackets were loading two couples onto a yellow and black tube tied behind a small speed boat. She could see the sun descending lazily toward the water. Every opportunity for fun, excitement, and romantic joy were available.

Available to everyone but me, she thought, staring down at her glass. She wondered what Marissa and Ethan were doing right now, how they were handling this entire situation. It was evident that the wedding was still happening. Sydney was sure that had been a difficult decision for them as a couple.

She sighed as she turned and walked back into the room. She carefully dressed herself in the sleeveless Carolina Herrera dress she had packed from Rent the Runway. The emerald green fabric cascaded over her curves in a mixture of ruffles and folds, and she caught a look at herself in the mirror. *Picture perfect*, she thought staring at her reflection. She wished the rest of her life fit as well as her dress.

"You look gorgeous," Alex said as he stepped into the room. Sydney turned around to face him and immediately blushed. He was standing at the edge of the bed, wrapped only in a towel. Beads of water from the shower trickled down his muscular physique. She stared a few extra seconds, in spite of herself.

"Thanks," she said, stumbling over her words. "I'll just finish my makeup while you get dressed."

She carefully applied her makeup, barely thinking through the steps as she concentrated on what to do once they reached the cocktail party. She needed to speak to Will, see his face for herself. Then she could decide if she believed he was truly capable of murder. As she hung a set of gold tasseled earrings on her ear lobes, Alex peeked into the bathroom.

"Ready to do this?" he said, giving her a reassuring smile.

She sprayed a bit of Chanel No. 5 on her neck, then turned back to him.

"Ready."

FOURTEEN
SYDNEY

SYDNEY COULD HEAR the sound of faint piano music drifting over the ocean waves as she and Alex ambled along an elegantly paved path toward the piano bar. The giant white arms of the bar's roofline loomed in the distance, a brightly lit oasis against the dark sky. The sun had officially settled in for the night, leaving the pathway to be lit only by a series of small luminaries. Alex stayed close by her side, brushing up against her arm as they walked. It seemed as if they were alone. She assumed the rest of the guests had most likely arrived at the party.

The crowd grew louder and more dense as they approached. Alex placed his hand on her back as they drew closer. She could see at least a hundred people milling about the space, carrying small cocktail and wine glasses. A group of people crowded around a large white piano on the east end of the bar that was elevated by a tiled platform. She could barely see the top of a piano player's tan fedora bobbing along to the loud music.

"Can I offer you a drink?" said a woman wearing a tight white tuxedo dress.

"I'll have a rum and Diet Coke," said Alex, turning to the women with a smile. "Sydney?"

"Same," she said, barely looking at the waitress as she scanned the room.

"I figured you were more of a champagne-only kind of girl," said Alex as the waitress walked away. Sydney turned to looked at him, curling up a corner of her mouth.

"You were wrong," she said.

Sydney wondered what other assumptions Alex had already made about her. She knew that many people had false assumptions about who she was. Some people would certainly have classified her as "high maintenance." But to her, it was part of a job.

Their drinks arrived moments later. She hooked an arm around Alex's.

"Let's walk around and see if we can find Will," she whispered in his ear. The music and the sounds of conversation boomed around them. The layout of the space made it easy to see everyone but difficult to hear. As she leaned into Alex, she could feel the heat from his body and smell the hotel soap on his skin.

Just as they were about to make a full loop around the bar, she heard the PA system crackle overhead.

"Hello everyone," said a familiar voice. She looked over people's heads and saw Ethan standing on a platform behind the piano. He was dressed in a beige sport coat, his dark brown hair carefully styled and his face freshly shaved. "I just wanted to take a moment to welcome all of you to the resort."

She saw Marissa standing next to him, looking anxious as he spoke. She fingered a small tissue in her hands, keeping her eyes steadily on Ethan. She was wearing a long champagne-colored gown that shimmered in the torch lights that flickered around the room.

Ethan cleared his throat. "As many of you have heard, there was a tragic accident on our way here to Jamaica." He took a breath. "Our dear friend Lizzy Ortez has passed away." He paused and reached an arm around Marissa, who leaned into him. A hush fell over the crowd, as all heads in the room turned to watch the couple. Marissa began to quickly dab her eyes with the tissue. "After a long discussion, we have decided to move forward with the wedding. We believe that's what Lizzy would have wanted."

He looked down at Marissa, who nodded her approval. "Lizzy was a beautiful soul, and we will miss her deeply." He waited, letting the sentiment sink in with the crowd. "She also loved a good party. So this weekend, we will not only be celebrating our wedding, but also celebrating the life of our dear friend."

Marissa shifted her stance, looking around the room as Ethan raised his glass. A server quickly approached them and handed a glass to her.

"So please raise your glasses and help us honor our dear friend." He raised his glass. "To Lizzy."

"To Lizzy," the crowd echoed.

Sydney and Alex joined the rest of the room and raised their glasses. After everyone had taken a collective drink, the piano music began to play. People returned to their conservations and their phones, feverishly talking and texting. She could practically see the news of Lizzy's death flooding the social media feeds.

Sydney wobbled a bit, a rush of emotions surging through her. Her eyes began to fill with tears as she thought of the collective sadness and shock people must be feeling. She wanted to find Marissa and hug her. Share the intense grief that they must both be feeling. But the less time Alex spent with Marissa and Ethan the better. There was enough suspicion surrounding them, and she was sure any conversation with Alex would only make things worse.

As she saw them step off the platform, she grabbed Alex's arm.

"Come on, we have to find Will," she said, leading him in the opposite direction of the couple.

The bar was set away from the resort, an oval island extending out into the beach. While the end of the bar closest to the resort was densely crowded, the other end was set farther out into the darkness of the beach. She could see a bleach-blonde leaning over a man at the bar. She instantly recognized the mousy-brown hair of Will Sauder.

With relief, she headed in his direction. She wasn't sure how she should be feeling in that moment. Anger toward Will? Sadness for him? She had to suspend any emotions until she knew the truth. As they came closer, she could already see he was in bad shape. His hair was matted down on his forehead, and he was wearing a white V-neck T-shirt splattered with stains. It was a sharp contrast to the cocktail attire of the rest of the partygoers. She could smell a mixture of booze and body odor within a few feet of his perch.

"Will?" she said, edging closer.

"Sydney?" he said, looking up at her. She could immediately see his eyes were bloodshot from a lack of sleep. "Sydney, it's Lizzy. She's...gone."

Sydney reached out and patted him on the shoulder. Perhaps a hug should have been in order, but she was sure Rent the Runway would not accept her dress back if she had any of what Will was wearing on it.

"I know, Will, I'm so sorry." She could barely hold back her own tears as she spoke. She took a deep breath and stood back, steadying herself. "Do you know what happened?"

Will looked down at his glass, which appeared to be a fresh cocktail of some sort with a lime hanging off the side. She guessed that the bartender didn't have the heart to cut him off yet.

"They said it was food poisonin'," he said, shaking his head. Sydney and Alex exchanged a look. "I don't get it. One minute she was fine, and then"—he shook his head harder—"she was gone."

Will was clearly drunk, and she started to wonder if her plans to sniff out his story were ill conceived. Sydney had to swallow hard as a lump of emotion began to form in her throat. Alex stepped in closer to her, placing a hand on her back. Will seemed to take note of him and peered up at him curiously.

"Who's this? Captain 'Merica?" he said, slurring.

"This is Alex. He is my date for the wedding."

"Huh," Will replied, squinting slightly. "Where's Jack?"

Sydney took a step back, tripping on the hem of her dress. Alex quickly reached over to steady her. It had been months since she had heard any of her friends speak Jack's name. She was sure Will was in shock, possibly forgetting that Jack was dead. Her heart began pumping at a fast pace as she felt the heat rise into her cheeks. It took every bit of willpower she could muster not to turn and run away that very moment.

Will pushed back his bar stool and tried to stand.

"No worries," he said. He stumbled, groping for the bar as he tried to regain his balance. His tall chair tipped back, knocking Will's feet from under him and sending him tumbling to the ground. Sydney thought she saw something fall out of his pocket as he fell.

Alex jumped into action, reaching down to pull Will back to his feet. The sudden jerking motion caused Will to lurch forward and vomit all over Alex's pants. Sydney took a few steps back, covering her mouth. To his credit, Alex kept his hands on Will's arm, continuing to steady him.

"Sorry, Captain," Will said, a look of embarrassment crossing his face.

"No worries," said Alex. Sydney saw him scan the area. He then nodded to two servers who were watching the entire scene. As they approached, Alex handed Will over to them.

"Make sure he gets back to his room," he said. They nodded.

Meanwhile, Sydney noticed the dark object that had fallen out of Will's pocket was lying on the ground. As Will stumbled away, she pulled up the hem of her long dress and reached down to pick it up.

What she held in her hand was a dark grey velvet box. She knew what small boxes of this size usually held. Her heart began to beat a little faster, and she pried open the lid. She let out a small gasp as Alex returned to her side.

"What is it?" he asked.

"An engagement ring."

They stood there next to each other at the end of the bar staring at the box. As the crowd chattered raucously around them, they stood quietly, as if having a moment of silence for a wedding that would never be.

"Oh, Lizzy," she said breathlessly, staring at the ring. "She would have been so happy." The last words came out almost as a whisper.

The pain of her past was now unavoidable. She had lost so many dreams of her own when Jack died. Now she had to accept the loss of her friend's dreams too. A wave of nausea hit her and she swayed. She didn't think she could bear another moment of the party.

"We need to go," she said, as she clipped the lid shut on the box. "Here, take this. We can return it to Will later." She thrust the small box toward him.

"I think you're right," he said, pocketing the box into his stained pants.

As the two of them made their way to the beachside path that lead back to the hotel, Sydney began to put together what had happened. If Will was truly set to propose to her friend, surely he wouldn't have wanted to kill her. He obviously had plans for their future, not to mention the state of grief he was in seemed genuine. The thought made her sad, as she knew Lizzy had always wanted to settle down and raise a family.

Alex kept his arm around her and they walked briskly down the path. She was too exhausted to pretend she didn't need the support right now. She could see the sprawling hotel up ahead and tried to focus on the silky soft bed sheets that awaited her arrival. She wanted to close her eyes and make it all go away.

But one question continued to burn intensely in her mind.

If Will didn't kill Lizzy, who did?

FIFTEEN
ETHAN

THE NEXT MORNING Ethan arrived back at the hotel with two arms full of paper gift bags, bursting with brightly colored tissue paper. He had spent the morning at Montego Bay running errands and picking out gifts for his future wife. Although it was only late morning, the heat from the sun was already causing him to sweat through his clothing. As soon as he walked back through the white archways of the hotel, he pulled a small box out of one of the bags and handed the rest over to a bellman. He then set his eyes on the lobby bar.

He hooked his sunglasses into his pale blue shirt and sat down on a leather upholstered bar stool partly facing the ocean. He placed the box on the countertop next to him. The smell of Jamaican jerk chicken wafted over the bar— the restaurant next door was preparing for lunch. He could hear the clanging of silverware as the hotel chef barked orders at his staff.

"What can I get for ya?" asked the bartender, tossing a white bar towel over his shoulder as he walked down to Ethan's perch.

"Double scotch, Dewar's, on the rocks."

"Yeah, man." The dark-skinned bartender nodded and strolled back to his row of liquors. There was one couple at the far end of the bar who looked like they had just returned from the pool. Other than that, the bar was fairly empty. Ethan's phone began to vibrate. He pulled it out of his linen pants and glanced down at the number. He had two text message notifications.

He read the first message that popped up, which came from his secretary, Alice.

Documents are ready. I'll have them with me when I see you later.

Ethan nodded to himself, quickly typing a response. *And there is no trace of what happened? Nothing to raise any suspicion?*

Everything is perfect, she typed back a few moments later. *Just as we discussed.*

Thanks Alice, you are a life saver.

Anything for you my dear, she responded.

The bartender returned with his scotch. Ethan took a long drink, staring thoughtfully at the back of the bar. He knew Alice would do anything to protect him. She had been like a second mother to him and Jack. The only person in his life, other than his brother, he felt like he could trust.

"You the man who's getting married tomorrow?" asked the bartender, interrupting his thoughts.

Ethan took another swig of his glass. "So they tell me."

"I've seen you with the lady—she is a beauty. You are a lucky man."

Ethan finished his glass. "Yeah, lucky," he said, staring at the bottom of the glass. "I'll have another."

He *had* felt lucky when he met Marissa. She was beautiful, smart, and incredibly wealthy. Unlike many of the rich business-tycoon types he dealt with, where ego was king, Marissa handled her wealth with grace and humility. Marrying her didn't just mean landing the catch of the decade; it was also a direct reflection of his own success. They would make a powerful pair.

As he drained his second glass, he noted an unread message from an unknown number. He knew it was from his private investigator, Derrick Bishop. He had hired Bishop to make sure Sydney didn't cause any problems at the wedding. Knowing she was in a fragile state, Ethan worried she wouldn't show up. Ethan knew that if Sydney didn't show, Marissa would call off the wedding. They were already on shaky ground after the incident on the plane.

He peered down at his phone.

She's arrived on the island, the message read. *A man came with her. He looks like former military. Possibly a fed.*

Was she at the party last night? Ethan texted back. He had heard a few whispers that she had showed up but had not seen her himself. He was too busy managing the entire ordeal around Lizzy's death, not to mention Marissa, who was understandably distraught the whole night.

Yes. She was with the man. They spoke to Will Sauder and left.

Ethan tapped a finger against his glass. Will seemed pretty harmless, but he needed to be handled carefully.

Keep following her. Be careful, if her date is a fed, he'll spot you from a mile away.

Don't worry man, I got this.

Suddenly, he felt a soft hand work its way down his shoulder. Ethan nearly jumped out of his bar seat.

"Ethan!" Marissa said, looking perplexed as she leaned in and gave him a kiss. "Where have you been all morning? I couldn't find you anywhere."

He quickly put down his phone, darkening the screen before she could catch sight of his messages.

"I'm sorry, I was just out running a few errands."

"We had a meeting with Jessica this morning at nine. Did you forget?" She furrowed her perfectly drawn brows at him looking irritated.

"Oh no, I forgot," he said as he tapped his hand to his forehead, emphasizing the point. "I hope you were able to get through it without me. I trust Jessica is still doing a good job?"

Ethan reached over and brushed a long strand of auburn hair off her shoulders. She was wearing a navy-blue jumpsuit that fell off her shoulders and highlighted her bronzed skin. He could smell the jasmine oil in her hair mixed with some expensive perfume. She gave him a pouty look, then settled back into her seat.

"Yes, she's doing fine. But I would have liked to have you there." She paused and looked off toward the beach. He could see the stress of everything was beginning to weigh on her.

"I suppose I'm a little on edge," she said, playing with her cocktail napkin. "With everything that's happened."

Ethan rubbed her shoulder. "I know, babe. It's hard. We'll get through it, I promise." He reached over and slid a box in front of her.

"Look, I brought you something."

He could see her eyes brighten at the sight of the small oblong box that was tied with a matching grey velvet ribbon. She reached for it and carefully untied the ribbon, balancing the box in her hand. As she pulled open the hinged lid, her eyes sparkled.

"Oh, Ethan, it's beautiful."

Ethan watched as she pulled a large diamond tennis

bracelet out. Ethan had spent a fortune on the bracelet, quickly picking it out at an expensive boutique in Kingston called Joyaux des Iles. The shop was by appointment only, and he had called in a few favors to have them open up early. The sales associate had nearly giggled with joy as she wrapped it up for him. He was always amazed at the effects that diamonds had on women. In this case, it was the perfect way to win some goodwill with his emotionally fragile fiancée.

"Thank you," she whispered and leaned in to give him a kiss.

"Only the best for you," he said, helping her place the bracelet on her wrist. She smiled as she touched it lightly with the opposite hand.

"Listen, I have to run to another meeting. I'll see you tonight before the rehearsal dinner?" she said, looking slightly teary-eyed.

"Of course. I love you, Marissa."

"Love you too," she said.

Ethan watched her as she walked away, her long auburn hair swaying like a river down her back, the bracelet sparkling in the tropical sun. As soon as she was out of sight, Ethan reached down and felt for the thin folded piece of paper in his pocket.

Joyaux des Iles had a strict policy about returning items without a receipt.

SIXTEEN

SYDNEY

SYDNEY AWOKE to a quiet but insistent knock on the door. She pulled her silk sleep mask up above her face and glared in that direction. The room was still dark but only because she had hastily pulled the heavy polyester curtains shut before passing out in her bed. She had slept deeply after taking another Ambien.

The door thumped again. She looked over to the sofa bed and saw Alex sleeping soundly in a T-shirt and boxer shorts. He looked sort of peaceful. His skin had a tiny bit of glow from their first day in Jamaica. His long brown eyelashes cast a small shadow over his cheeks. She wondered if he had fallen asleep right after her.

As she stood up and reached for her floral silk robe, a generous welcome gift from Marissa, the unsettling notion that they still had no solid leads in Lizzy's murder returned. She swayed a bit before stumbling toward the door then pulling it open to find Maxwell with his ever-present smile.

"Good morning, madam. I am so sorry to wake you, but the pants for Mr. Alex are ready," he said holding up a wooden hanger with the pants neatly folded over the side. "I thought he might need them for today?"

"Yes, thank you," she replied, taking the hanger and tossing it on the large bed. She was impressed with how quickly they had handled his dry cleaning. She was sure it wasn't the first time something like that had happened at the resort.

"I also brought you some fresh coffee and breakfast."

She peered behind Maxwell and saw a small table with two silver domes. Coffee, orange juice, and bowls of fruit were carefully wrapped in plastic for freshness.

"Yes, thank you, Maxwell. You are amazing."

"My pleasure," he said with his thick Jamaican accent. As he pushed the cart into the room, Sydney stashed the bag in the closet. She turned around and watched Maxwell carefully place the two silver domes and the rest of the breakfast spread onto the small table. She noticed him eyeing Alex, asleep in the corner.

"We, uh, had a fight last night," Sydney said quickly, gesturing toward Alex. "You know, just a lovers' quarrel." She laughed nervously, trying to maneuver between Maxwell and the bed.

"Ah," Maxwell responded with a wry smile. "Maybe I can help. I could set up a nice couple's massage for you on the beach later today? To help you both relax?"

"Oh, no, that won't be necessary," Sydney said, walking Maxwell to the door. "I'm sure we will talk it out, um, over breakfast."

"Trust me, I have just the thing," he said.

"Really, it's fine," she said nearly pushing him out of the room. She heard Alex stir behind her and turned to see him sitting up in his makeshift bed.

"Is that coffee I smell?" he said, rubbing fresh stubble on the side of his cheek.

"It is," she said with a smile. Sydney pulled back the two silver domes to reveal a full suite of breakfast staples including eggs, bacon and fresh croissants. Her stomach grumbled as the steam rose from the plates. She suddenly found her appetite again. "And breakfast. You hungry?"

"Always." He grabbed a pair of plaid pajama pants heaped next to the sofa. He pulled them on, stretched, and shuffled over to her at the small table, which was now set up for a cozy breakfast for two. Before sitting down, he reached over and carefully poured two cups of coffee from a silver carafe.

The whole setting felt quite intimate, and Sydney grew nervous. She reached for her phone, a welcome distraction to her anxiousness.

"Wait, I want to get a photo," she said. She quickly pushed a few plates around, folded a napkin and stashed it under a corner of one plate, and rearranged the coffee cups. She made sure to leave Alex's cup out of the photo. She then pulled the hem of her robe and stood on the chair to get an overhead view of their breakfast spread.

"That looks dangerous," Alex said, staring up at her curiously.

"I do it all the time." She took about twenty rapid-fire photos before stepping down onto the floor. "Part of the job, I guess."

"I see," he said nodding his chin in her direction. "May I eat now?"

Sydney noted his sarcastic tone and was instantly irritated. She settled back into her seat and glared at him as she picked up a steaming cup of coffee. "You may."

Alex grabbed a plate of bacon and eggs and pulled it to his side of the table. "Does it ever get old, you know, documenting every moment of your life? Making everything look perfect?"

Sydney narrowed her eyes at him as she took a few sips of her coffee. "I don't try to make everything look *perfect*. I just try to make things look, you know, better than they would in everyday life." She reached for a slice of bacon. "People like to be inspired."

"I see."

"You wouldn't understand."

"Probably not."

Sydney sighed and added a few more items to her plate. She had always been a nervous eater and Alex wasn't helping. He had hit a nerve with her about her life, but she wasn't quite ready to face it. She decided to redirect the conversation to more urgent matters.

"So clearly Will is not our guy," she said looking over at Alex as he poured himself another cup of coffee.

"I don't think so. I spoke to some of my guys last night after you passed out."

Sydney looked down at her coffee, slightly embarrassed. "Will has done pretty well for himself financially and doesn't need the money. Not to mention the engagement ring."

"So now what?" she said, looking over at him.

Alex shrugged. "Well, I'm afraid Marissa and Ethan—"

"No, I know it's not them," she said, straightening up in her chair. "There has to be someone we've overlooked."

"Who else knew that Lizzy would be on the plane?"

Sydney went through a mental checklist of everyone in Marissa and Ethan's entourage. Marissa had a bubbly personal assistant named Evie, but she was young and harmless. Ethan had about fifty employees who worked in his office. He kept most of them at arm's length, and many hadn't even been invited to the wedding.

She suddenly remembered that Lizzy had told her she had started a job at his office a few months ago. Sydney had distanced herself from Lizzy a bit after the news; anything that had to do with Ethan and Jack's company brought with it too much pain. But from what she remembered, Lizzy had been working under Ethan's secretary.

"Alice," Sydney said, spilling a bit of her coffee as she set it down on the table.

"The secretary?"

"Yes, Ethan and Alice were very close. She handled all his travel plans, personal details as well as managing their office. She would have had access to their entire itinerary. Plus, she worked with Lizzy."

Alex cocked his head as she spoke, clearly considering what she had to say.

"Okay, I'll play along. Why would Alice want to have Lizzy poisoned?"

"Alice was very protective of Ethan and Jack." She swallowed as she said his name. "When the boys were teenagers, their parents passed away. They had to be placed into foster care for several years before they were old enough to go out on their own." She pulled her robe on a little tight, feeling the air-conditioning kick on in the room. "Alice was their last foster mom."

"I see," said Alex, leaning in. "But that still doesn't give Alice a motive for murder."

Sydney pulled a few strands of her hair through her fingers, thinking for a moment. "I remember when Lizzy started working with Alice. They didn't really get along. She said that Alice was very uptight around her. She was also shooing her out of her office. Lizzy was frustrated because she couldn't get Alice to let her do anything except organize office supplies and go for coffee. She said she thought Alice was hiding something."

Alex seemed to perk up at this, setting his own coffee down on the table. "What was she hiding?"

"I don't know," Sydney said, staring off toward the window. "We were supposed to get together and catch up before the wedding, but..." She felt her eyes well up with tears. "I guess I was avoiding her. Hearing about her work at Jack's old company was too painful for me."

"I get it," said Alex, nodding.

She brushed her fingertips against the bottom of her eyelids, refusing to let herself fall apart. "But if she found out something she shouldn't have..." She paused, looking directly at Alex. "Then maybe Alice wanted to keep her quiet. Permanently."

As she thought about the notion, she felt a sense of anger well up inside of her. Sweet Lizzy, who never would have harmed a fly. How could someone have taken advantage of her like that? If it was possible that Alice had anything to do with her death, Sydney would do everything she could to bring her to justice.

"Sydney, I think you might be on to something," Alex said as he stood up. "I'll make a few calls. In the meantime, you do whatever it is you do to get ready," he said, looking her up and down with a slight smile. "And then we can go have a chat with Alice the secretary."

Although slightly offended by his tone, Sydney was elated that he had accepted her theory. She might very well be wrong about Alice, but at the very least, it took the heat off Marissa and Ethan.

"Sounds like a plan, Agent Birch," she said sarcastically. Then, without much thought, she grabbed the pair of freshly cleaned pants off the bed and hurled them at Alex's head.

"And by the way, your pants are clean."

SEVENTEEN

SYDNEY

AN HOUR LATER, Sydney and Alex stepped into the main lobby of the hotel. The large domed ceiling hung overhead, with a patchwork of weathered wood beams that seemed to wrap their arms languidly around the guests below. The sounds of rolling suitcases, high-heeled shoes, and giant brass carts bounced off the walls and filled the room with a hum that rivaled the Jamaican band playing outside on the beach. Many of the guests were couples, huddled together or holding hands as they walked. Sydney found herself feeling suddenly lonely, even though Alex never kept but a few inches from her elbow.

She had been careful to dress herself modestly, wearing a plain beige linen dress. She had tied her long hair into a side braid and donned a panama-style hat and sunglasses to conceal her face. The last thing she needed was for someone to spot her and try to speak to her about Lizzy. Alex had quickly pulled on a navy T-shirt and khaki shorts, which actually suited him.

She spotted the concierge sign above a massive

mahogany desk, just to the left of the main hotel entrance. Alex kept close to her as they made their way in that direction. Sydney nearly tripped over a bellman who was scurrying past with a cart full of Louis Vuitton luggage as she approached the stand.

"Hello...Alvita," said Sydney, taking off her glasses for a moment so she could read the name badge hanging from the woman's chest. She looked as if she was in her fifties, a beautiful black Jamaican with thick salt-and-pepper braids woven in a halo around her head. She was dressed head to toe in an all-white uniform, matching the rest of the hotel staff who bustled around the room. "I was hoping you could help me. I am looking for a close friend of mine who is arriving for the wedding today. Her name is Alice Mitchell."

"Yes, ma'am. I would be happy to help you," she said with a wide grin. "What is your name and room number?"

"Sydney Evans." She cleared her throat and nearly whispered, "Honeymoon suite number five."

The woman seemed to perk up at this news.

"Aw, yes, Mrs. Evans! We hope you are enjoying your beautiful room and everything it has to offer." As she said this, she raised her eyebrows at Alex, who was standing close to Sydney. Alex pursed his lips, trying not to laugh. Alvita looked down at her computer and quickly began typing. "I trust Maxwell is taking good care of you?"

"Yes, he's been great. Now could we—"

"Oh," said the woman, raising her eyebrows, "I see he has booked you a couple's massage on the beach." She peered up at Sydney. "I have heard we may have a bit of rain this afternoon. How about I move you to our special couple's massage room in the Serendipity Spa?"

"No, really that's okay, we—"

"Oh, don't be shy, Mrs. Evans. It's important to take advantage of this time you have together as a couple." She smiled. "It's *very* romantic."

"We can't—"

"Please, you will enjoy it so much," she said, her eyes full of earnest joy. Sydney could hardly say no to this very persuasive and enthusiastic Jamaican woman.

"Okay, fine." She gave Alex a sideways look, daring him to speak. He had a slight smirk on his face but simply shrugged in response. "We will be there."

She looked back at Alvita. "Now, can you tell me if Alice Mitchell has arrived for the wedding?"

"I'm sorry, Mrs. Evans, it is strictly against our policy to share the names of our guests and room numbers," she said. Sydney's face dropped, but Alvita continued undeterred. "I'm sure that Miss Mitchell will be at the rehearsal dinner party this evening, perhaps you can catch up with her then?"

"But, you see, Alvita, it's urgent that I speak with her, today."

"I'm so sorry," she said. "We have a very strict policy."

"But—"

"Now, you have just enough time for a quick stroll on the beach or perhaps a casual lunch at our delicious buffet before your massage. Would you like me to give you directions?"

Sydney's shoulders slumped. "No, we're fine."

"Wonderful. Enjoy your massage."

Sydney stormed away from the desk, pushing her sunglasses back onto her face. She couldn't be upset with Alvita, but it was all she could do to remain polite. Apparently finding Alice was going to be a bit harder than she had anticipated. Just as she was about to tell Alex they needed to head back to the room to regroup, she heard a woman's voice boom across the room.

"Sydney!" cried Marissa coming toward her. Sydney felt a rush of relief and panic as her friend hurried in her direction. Before she could muster a response, Marissa had wrapped her arms around her in a cloud of Guerlain perfume.

"Marissa, I'm so happy to see you," she said, nearly gasping for breath. As Marissa held on to her, she made eye contact with Alex. He silently mouthed the words *introduce me*. Sydney rolled her eyes at him. As she pulled back, Sydney held Marissa's hands in her own. "How are you holding up?"

"Oh, you know, it's been hard," said Marissa, swallowing deeply. "But I know Lizzy would have wanted us to go through with the wedding. She was so...happy for us." Marissa's eyes began to look glassy as she spoke. Sydney grasped her hands a little harder.

"You're doing the right thing, Marissa," she said.

Marissa threw her arms around her again. "Oh Sydney, I'm so glad you are here." She pulled away from her and said, "Listen, I've got to run to another meeting. Can we catch up tonight after the rehearsal? I've really missed you."

"Of course," said Sydney smiling at her.

"Great, I'll see you then," she said. Marissa turned and walked briskly toward the north end of the hotel. Alex stepped closer to Sydney's side.

"Did she just completely ignore me?" he said, looking indignant.

Sydney nearly laughed. "Marissa has a way of sweeping in and sweeping out. Don't worry, I'll make sure to introduce you tonight." If Sydney was being honest, she was relieved that Alex hadn't had a chance to speak with Marissa yet; she was sure he would cause trouble.

"So how are we going to find Alice now?" Alex didn't seem to be paying attention to her. He appeared to be looking over her shoulder. She followed his gaze across the room.

"Maxwell," he said, walking toward the front desk. The tall butler turned around and gave him a puzzled look but then quickly walked to meet him. Sydney tagged along behind.

"I was hoping you could help me with something."

"Of course, sir. What is it?" he said, his eyes gleaming with sincerity.

"Well, I'm trying to track down a friend of Sydney's, but we are having trouble finding her room."

"I'm sorry sir; we have a strict policy—"

"So I've heard. Listen." Alex then pulled out what looked like a rolled-up hundred-dollar bill and passed it over to the white-gloved butler. "I will make it worth your while. Her name is Alice Mitchell. You give us her room number and no one has to know."

"I see," said Maxwell as he pocketed the bill. "I'll make you an even better deal, Mr. Birch. If you and your lovely girlfriend will show up for the couple's massage I have booked for you, I will meet you with the information afterward." He looked back and forth between them and lowered his voice. "You see, it makes me look good to my boss if my guests are having a good time."

"Maxwell, you have a deal. We'll see you later."

Maxwell gave them a curt nod and then turned and walked away.

"Nicely done," said Sydney, smiling at Alex. "But getting a massage is the last thing I need right now."

Alex shrugged. "You never know. You might think better when you're relaxed."

"I'll take your word for it," she replied.

EIGHTEEN
SYDNEY

THE INTOXICATING SMELLS of eucalyptus and lavender washed over Sydney as she lay silently on a soft white massage table in a large rectangular room dimly lit with candles and covered in rose petals. Two female massage therapists had pushed, pulled, and kneaded the knots in her back as she lay facing Alex on the table. She could feel a little bit of drool puddle at the corner of her mouth as she felt the tension leave her body. Maybe Maxwell had been right about his suggestion of a massage, as it felt long overdue.

Of course, a few moments earlier, she hadn't quite felt so relaxed when she and Alex had arrived wearing white cotton robes and were instructed to undress and get comfortable. Alex had behaved as a gentleman, looking away while she disrobed and slid quickly under her sheet. There were two glasses of champagne waiting for them, along with freshly cut strawberries. After Sydney had donned her robe, she had taken a long drink of her champagne, hoping it would help take the edge off.

As the masseuse prodded her with skilled hands, she let

her thoughts wander to any memories she had of Alice. She met Alice shortly after she and Jack had begun dating. Sydney had come to the DoubleDownCasino.com office in downtown Chicago to surprise him for lunch.

Of course, she had picked the worst day. It was pouring rain, the L train had broken down, and she had to walk three blocks without an umbrella to reach his office. By the time she got there, she was soaked through, her hair rivaling the look of a wet rat. Determined to keep going, she stopped into the lobby restroom and managed to put herself back together. By the time she reached the front desk of the office, she was freshly powdered, combed, and perfumed.

Her newfound gumption was quickly dashed when she met the eyes of Alice Mitchell. A plump woman in her fifties, Alice wore her hair swept up in a tight bun. It was so tight, just looking at it gave Sydney a headache. She wore minimal makeup and kept her blue eyes hidden behind a pair of thick brown glasses. She straightened as Sydney walked into the room and put a forced smile on her face.

"Hello. How may I help you?"

Sydney felt nervous, like she was being reprimanded by her third grade teacher.

"Hi. I am here to meet Jack Evans?"

Alice peered at her. "I see. Do you have an appointment with Mr. Evans?"

"Well, no," she said, fumbling with the hem of her sweater. "I was going to surprise him."

Alice raised an eyebrow at her, rubbing her fingers around a small key that hung around her neck. Sydney stood there awkwardly, unsure what to do next. She thought about sending him a quick text or perhaps returning to the main floor to call him from the lobby. As she ran through a list of ideas, a tall figure passed through the glass hallway behind Alice's front entry desk.

A few seconds later, Jack burst through the door. He rushed to her side, picking her up and swinging her around like they hadn't seen each other in years. She saw Alice, out of the corner of her eye, lean down and quickly shut and lock a filing cabinet drawer next to her desk.

"Sydney!" he said as a wide smile broke across his face. "What are you doing here?"

"I wanted to surprise you," she said giving him a quick kiss on the cheek.

Alice stood like a statue behind the desk, staring at the both of them.

"Oh, I'm sorry Alice. Have you met Sydney?"

"Briefly," she responded, mustering up a pleasant enough smile.

"Sydney, this is Alice. She is an old friend and our secretary here at the office."

Alice seemed to glow under his gaze, giving him a much warmer smile in return. Sydney learned later on that Alice was much more than a secretary. She had known the twins since they were teenagers and had stuck with them since then, filling the role of a second mother to them.

After that day, Alice had always made an effort to be pleasant with her when she came to visit the office, but it felt forced. She sensed that Alice was possessive of the twins and wondered if she was jealous of her close relationship with Jack. The key she wore around her neck was always present. Sydney thought it a bit old-school but didn't give it much thought after that.

But now it seemed relevant. Lizzy, in the brief conversations they'd had since she started working at Ethan's office, had mentioned the key several times. She asked Sydney if she thought it was odd they way Alice always kept her desk drawer locked and actually wore the key around her neck. Lizzy had even suggested she might take the key one night and finally find out what she kept hidden in her desk.

Maybe she found out Alice's secret, Sydney thought as the masseuse gently laid the towel over her back. The soft instrumental music continued to play throughout the room. Sydney felt sleepy and had to force herself to open her eyes again. It was her newfound determination to speak with Alice that woke her up.

As her eyes began to flutter open, she realized she was still facing Alex, who lay still on the table across from her. They both must have fallen asleep during the massage, exhausted from the day before.

As her eyes began to focus, she realized there was a figure leaning over him. She noticed that the masseur, however, was not wearing the traditional white uniform. He was wearing all black. As her brain tried to place his odd appearance, her eyes caught a beam of light reflect off an object in the man's hand. He was holding a large syringe, pointing it directly at Alex's neck.

As a bolt of adrenaline seized her heart, she opened her mouth to scream but nothing came out. It was like a nightmare where you couldn't speak.

Alex! she tried to say and failed.

A moment later, she found her voice. As loud as she could muster, she screamed, "Alex! Wake up!"

The man in black looked up at her, startled. Alex's eyes burst open, and he immediately jumped up from the table, knocking the man off balance. The silver syringe clattered to the ground. Sydney laid frozen for a moment, watching the two of them struggle. She jumped up and grabbed her robe, quickly pulling it on. The man in black lunged for the door.

Alex, dressed only in his underwear, caught the man by the back of his neck.

As the man swung around to face him, Alex delivered a powerful punch to his face. The man cried out in pain and grabbed his nose. Blood burst from his nose, soaking his clothes and splattering all over the carpet. Alex took the opportunity to grab the man's arm and wrestle him down to the ground.

Moments later, the man was pinned, with his stomach on the floor. As he squirmed, Alex wrapped the man's arms behind him and straddled his back. He held him there while he leaned down and spoke in the man's ear.

"Why are you here?" he said, nearly spitting on him as he spoke. Alex was out of breath. She could see the sweat pouring down his back.

"No comprende, señor," replied the man in a thick Spanish accent.

"Oh, I think you understand," he said, twisting the man's arms harder. He cried out in pain as he writhed violently on the floor.

"I can't tell you," the man said in accented English. "They will kill me."

"Or I could do the job for them," said Alex. Just as he was about to twist the man's arms again, they heard a soft knock at the door.

"Mrs. Evans, Mr. Birch? Are you all right?" said Maxwell's muffled voice.

Alex looked at Sydney with raised eyebrows and gestured for her to speak.

"Uh, yes, Maxwell. We're great." She looked at Alex, eyes wide. "I will be right out!"

"Wonderful," he said. "I will wait here."

She looked at Alex. "What now?" she said in a loud whisper.

"Quick, grab the belt from my robe and throw it to me," he said. The man started shouting, and Alex shoved his hand over his mouth. Sydney ran to the other side of the room and yanked the belt from his robe. As she walked back to hand it to him, Alex said, "I need yours too."

"But—"

"I won't look, I promise" he said. She pulled the belt from her own robe and handed both to him. As she watched, Alex made quick work of tying the man's hands behind his back. He took the other belt and used it to gag him. Sydney was impressed with how quickly and deftly he handled the entire situation. It was clearly not his first time wrestling someone to the ground.

"What do we do now?" she whispered. She looked around the room for the massage therapists but they were gone.

"Grab my phone from the pocket of my shorts and bring it over to me," he said, gesturing to his clothes that were hanging on a hook next to the door.

She did so, tip-toeing around the room. Alex sat patiently on top of the man as the blood oozed out from his nose onto the floor. Sydney handed him the phone and then stood back and wrapped the robe tightly around herself.

"I'm going to get my guys in here to clean up this mess," he said, gesturing to the man underneath him. "I need you to go with Maxwell and cover for me."

"What about Alice?" she asked, shifting her weight inside the plush robe.

"Go to her room and see if you can find anything. But, Sydney"—he looked directly into her eyes, his own grey eyes sparkling with intensity—"please be careful."

Sydney looked at the man on the floor, who moments ago was holding a needle over Alex's neck. She looked back at Alex, her heart pounding as she nodded. "I'll try."

Sydney quickly walked to the hook on the other side of the door, grabbed her clothes and purse, and held them to her chest. As she reached for the handle of the door, Alex stopped her.

"Oh, and Sydney," he said.

"Yes?"

"Thanks for waking me up. I think you saved me from a painful afternoon," he said, a slight smile on his face as he gestured to the needle of the floor.

Sydney smiled back, in spite of herself.

"No problem," she said and quickly stepped out the door.

NINETEEN

SYDNEY

"MRS. EVANS, IS EVERYTHING ALL RIGHT?" Maxwell said in a hushed tone. His concern was evident by the deep creases in his aged forehead.

Sydney's heart was still beating wildly after the events in the massage room. She had quickly closed the heavy door behind her. Just outside it was a long hallway with brightly colored plush carpeting, designed to dampen any noise that might disturb the patrons of the spa. Hopefully there was enough insulation in the walls that no one had heard the scuffle inside.

"Yes, Maxwell, everything is fine. Alex, um, needed a little more time to get dressed." She hoped that her nervous tone did not betray her. "Were you able to find out the room number of my friend, Alice?"

Maxwell studied her for a moment, as if deciding whether or not to ask more questions. Sydney stood silently, waiting. She knew it was the nature of his job to show discretion for his guests, and quite frankly, she was banking on it.

"Yes," he said and slipped her a small sheet of paper.

Sydney quickly unfolded the paper with one hand and saw a room number written inside. "My coworkers tell me she arrived a few hours ago."

"Thank you Maxwell. I appreciate your help."

"It is my pleasure to serve you in any way I can," he responded with an informal bow.

Sydney smiled back and began to walk around him to the exit of the spa building. Just as she was a few steps away, she stopped and looked back at him. "Maxwell, can I ask you something?"

"Yes, ma'am?"

"Do you know Alvita, the older woman who works at the concierge?" she said. It had just occurred to her that Alvita was the person who had switched her and Alex to the "special room." She wondered if the woman had tipped off their attacker.

Maxwell gave her a puzzled look. "I'm sorry, Mrs. Evans. There is no Alvita who works in Concierge."

"But I spoke with her this morning; she booked us this room at the spa."

Maxwell frowned again. "I have worked at this resort for over ten years. I know everyone from the bellman to the line cook. I would remember a woman named Alvita."

Sydney felt butterflies in her stomach. She wondered why anyone would have wanted to lead them here, and attack Alex. She realized she was staring at Maxwell, and quickly recovered.

"Oh, I'm sorry. I must have misremembered her name," she said, adding a nervous laugh. "I better get going. Thanks again!"

She turned and walked quickly down the hallway before the elderly butler could ask her any more questions. She stopped in the women's locker room on her way, changing out of her robe and into regular clothes. The back of her linen dress clung to the thick lotion the masseuse had rubbed onto her skin.

She still couldn't believe what had just happened. She wondered how long it would take for Alex's team to show up and carry the black-clad Latin man away. She guessed he was up for a long afternoon chatting with the feds.

She sat down on the long wooden bench that ran parallel to the wall of oak-paneled lockers. It was logical to assume that the intentionally blown tire and the spa room attack were somehow related. But were those events related to Lizzy's death? While it was somewhat plausible to believe that Alice the cantankerous secretary would have Lizzy murdered to hide some secret, it seemed impossible that she was some dangerous criminal mastermind.

Sydney again unfolded the piece of paper that Maxwell had given her and read the room scrawled across the paper: 2271 Azul Terrace. She knew the Azul Terrace section was on the south side of the resort, away from where she and Alex were staying. She guessed it was more the singles' side of the sprawling hotel.

She tucked it back into her nude-colored Gucci purse, stood up, and walked out into the hallway. If Alice was hiding something, she had a better chance of discovering her secret before she talked to her. Sneaking into Alice's room therefore seemed to be the logical next step. She quickly exited the spa lobby and headed across the resort.

About ten minutes later, Sydney arrived at the elegantly carved wooden doorway of room 2271. She knocked a few times on the door, but no one responded. She realized that in her haste to find the room, she hadn't really put together a plan of how she was going to get inside. She stood there for a few minutes, trying to decide what to do next.

The sound of wheels squeaking down the hallway gave her an idea. On her way, she had passed a maid pushing a large cart of white towels, stopping at each room to replenish their supply. Sydney quickly retraced her steps and found the woman standing just around the corner.

"Oh, hello!" she said, giving the women her best smile. "You are just in time. I am completely out of towels already! Could you bring some to my room?"

"Of course, ma'am," she said eagerly. "What room are you in?"

"I'm in 2271, just around the corner," said Sydney, feeling emboldened. "I could use about ten towels or so. If that's okay?"

"Of course," she said. The woman grabbed a large stack of towels and followed Sydney back toward the room. As they approached, Sydney made a gasping sound.

"Oh no, I just stepped out and forgot my key." She wheeled around and looked helplessly at the woman. "Could you let me in?"

Sydney felt a little guilty for lying to this innocent women, whom she knew could get fired for what she was about to do. But if getting into Alice's room got her one step closer to understanding the mess she was in, then so be it.

The maid looked a bit uncomfortable. She shifted the heavy weight of the towels in her arms for a few seconds before nodding.

"No problem, ma'am," she said.

"I'll hold these," Sydney said as she reached over and grabbed the stack of towels from her arms.

A few moments later, Sydney stood inside Alice's room. The room was simple yet elegantly decorated with a large teal upholstered bed and soft grey walls. She looked around and saw a dark purple suitcase, which stood unopened next to the cabinet under the TV. There was a seating area next to the sliding glass doors facing the ocean with a small round table and two blue cushioned chairs. She spotted a black leather Tumi shoulder bag and small silver laptop sitting on the table.

She quickly strode across the room and sat down at the seat where Alice must have been sitting not long ago. She figured the computer would be locked, so she decided to dig into the bag. She pulled out a passport and various other travel documents, a silk pashmina, and a sleeping mask. There were a few yellow folders but nothing inside that she found interesting. After she had rifled through each pocket, she spread out all the pieces on the glossy wood tabletop next to the computer.

Nothing. Nothing stood out or created suspicion. Sydney sighed. She thought back to the locked cabinet in Double-DownCasino.com's Chicago office. *If there was something that important inside it, would Alice bring it with her?* she wondered.

She had featured a Tumi luggage set on her Instagram feed about seven months ago. The company had sent her an entire matching set with a bag similar to the one Alice had. It occurred to her that she hadn't searched the hidden travel pocket tucked inside the laptop slot. She decided to go back into the case and check again. She felt through each pocket carefully until she finally came to a small zipper on the inside of the padded laptop slot. She could feel something bulging inside.

Bingo.

She carefully unzipped the pocket and reached down inside. She could feel a rather fat envelope with a metal clasp. She pulled it out, placed it flat on the table, and undid the clasp. She tugged at the contents, which eventually gave way and tumbled out onto the table.

As the papers fanned out, her eyes quickly went to two documents that looked like copies of birth certificates. She read the names: Robert Lexington and Gabe Lexington, both born in Concord, New Hampshire, on March 22, 1984.

Sydney stopped, her finger frozen over the dates of birth. She blinked her eyes several times and looked again. *What? That can't be right.*

She began shuffling frantically through the rest of the paperwork, a mixture of court documents, fingerprints, and other pieces of official material. Her mind was racing. *Was it possible?* She refused to let herself believe anything until she had proof. But a few moments later, when her hand felt a thicker, smaller piece of paper, she had it.

It was a photograph: two small boys standing with their mother and father.

Twins.

It didn't take her but a moment to realize that she was looking at a photograph of Ethan and Jack as kids. They looked to be about ten years old. Sydney felt as if her eyes were glued to the photo. She had never seen a picture of Jack before the age of twenty-four. When she had asked him why he didn't have photographs of his childhood around, he had told her the photos were lost when a storage unit he shared with Ethan had flooded. Smitten with Jack at the time, she had taken his answer at face value. Now she wondered if that was true.

The boys were casually dressed, as if they had just come from a picnic, wearing matching khaki shorts. It was even more difficult to tell the younger version of the twins apart, but while one boy had a sullen stare, the other was smiling. She instantly recognized the smiling twin as Jack. She could spot that smile anywhere. Their parents stood behind them, the mother with a protective hand on Jack's shoulder and the father with a rather serious look behind Ethan. She couldn't quite place the feeling of why, but it seemed like something was off in their family dynamic. Regardless, the photo was definitely a young Ethan and Jack.

With a shaking hand, she turned over the photograph. Scrawled in blue ink on the back read: *The Lexingtons. Bill, Elaine, Gabe, and Robert. 1994.*

Sydney sat back in her chair, a wave of shock coursing through her body.

Why did Jack lie to her? Why did he change his name? Sydney's mind flashed back to the moment they signed their marriage certificate. Jack had gone to the effort of bringing her birth certificate and his own. She had barely glanced at the paperwork as she eagerly signed the documents. The questions started flying across her mind fast and fierce. She couldn't stop to think about the answers, only questions. Endless questions.

She needed more facts. More information about why Jack would have kept something so important in his life a secret from her. She shuffled through the paperwork again trying to find anything that might give her a clue. Nothing shed any more light other than just the names.

She bit her lip and pulled out her phone. She typed *Robert and Gabe Lexington* into the Google search bar. She scrolled for a few moments, but nothing came up. Then she typed in their names along with *New Hampshire*. That's when she received several hits.

The top result burned bright on her screen.

Twins Go Missing in House Fire. Parents Found Dead.

She clicked on the link, which took her to a news story from the *Concord Chronicle*, May 21, 1998. In the photograph were the same faces she had seen just moments ago, only older. Ethan and Jack as teenagers. The photograph was of them smiling in a school photo. She scrolled down farther to see the charred remains of the house.

Jack's childhood home.

The article said that the house had been burned to the ground, although the source of the fire was uncertain. Both parents' bodies were found inside. The boys, however, were missing. A massive search was under way, but so far the authorities hadn't had any leads.

She went back to Google and typed in *Missing twins, Jack and Gabe Lexington*. There were a few relevant hits, stating only that the case went cold. The boys were never found.

Until now. Sydney stared at the pashmina scarf lying on the table in front of her. What was Alice's connection to all this? Did she help them escape, or was she just the keeper of their secret?

Sydney looked up across the room and saw a digital clock next to the bed. It was 3:40; she had been in the room for more than thirty minutes—she knew she was pushing her luck. She pulled out her phone and quickly took photos of all the paperwork that was in the envelope. Next, she carefully repacked all the papers and put them back into the envelope, sealing the clasp once again.

Just as she was packing away the pashmina into Alice's travel bag, she heard a voice in the hallway. Sydney jumped up, shoved the shawl back into Alice's bag, and ran to the balcony door. The voice outside grew louder.

She fumbled with the large glass sliding door, but it wouldn't budge. Her eyes darted back and forth, looking for the lock. She heard the voice stop and the beep of the door key. Sydney gave up on the sliding door and dashed a few feet across the room and into the closet. She had just enough time to close the closet door before the room's front door opened.

"Yes, that's perfect. Please deliver it to room 2271. Thank you." She heard Alice's voice bounce across the walls as she stepped into the room.

Sydney was standing inside a small closet as wooden hangers dangled just in front of her face and brushed against her shoulders. She was afraid if she made one small move, she would send the entire set of hangers crashing to the floor. Although her heart was pounding, she tried to focus on taking quiet breaths in and out of her nose.

She could hear Alice moving around the room, unpacking her clothes. Sydney's heartbeat pounded in her ears. The thought of Alice opening the closet to find her standing there was paralyzing. If Alice was willing to kill someone to protect her secrets, what would she do to Sydney?

She heard the swoosh of the bathroom door open, followed by the shower coming on. *Yes!* If Alice took a shower, that would give her just enough time to slip out the door unnoticed. She felt herself relax a bit, breathing out some of her anxiety. Just as she did this, her shoulder knocked one of the wooden hangers loose and it banged against another hanger creating a domino effect, just as she had feared. They clattered to the floor, banging against every surface in the small space as they went.

Shit!

"Hello?" said Alice suddenly. "Is someone there?"

Sydney began to panic. She could hear Alice walking around the room, pulling on curtains and opening doors. Sydney couldn't decide which was worse, Alice opening the door to find her, or just coming out on her own.

She took a deep breath and chose the latter.

The closet door slid open, and Sydney stepped outside. Alice was facing the front door, her back to Sydney. She wheeled around to look at her. She was already in a white bathrobe, her long brown hair streaked with gray as it hung down past her shoulders. Sydney noticed she had a black object in her hand and extended it toward her in a quick motion. It took a moment for Sydney's brain to register what it was.

Alice was holding a gun. And it was pointed directly at her.

"Alice, wait! It's me, Sydney!"

TWENTY

SYDNEY

AS A FASHION INFLUENCER, Sydney's job had required
her to travel all over the world, sometimes to places where
she had found herself in what she had considered danger.
There was a dark alley in Prague where she thought she was
being followed, or the time she ended up in the slums of Rio
de Janeiro. But never is there a moment so intense or
dangerous as when there is a gun pointed directly at you.
For Sydney, this was a first.

"Sydney?" said Alice. She faltered slightly but kept the
the gun aimed at her. "What are you doing in my closet?"

Sydney's mind screamed for her to turn and run, but she
stayed put. "I...um...I just needed to talk to you, privately."

Alice cocked her head, considering this. After several
terrifying moments, she lowered the gun. "I'm sorry," she
said. "I should have lowered my gun as soon as I saw you."
Her eyes went to the floor. "I've been a little on edge lately."

"I know the feeling," Sydney said, finally allowing
herself to exhale. "Would you mind if we sat down for a
moment?"

"Sure," said Alice. She tightened the robe around her

waist, and the women took a seat across from each other. Alice placed the gun on the table between them. "What can I do for you, Sydney?"

Sydney considered her options. Did she just come out and ask her if she killed Lizzy? Did she ask her why she was hiding the twins' identities? Did she play a cat-and-mouse game of questions, or just go for the truth? As the options ran across her mind like ticker tape, Alice watched her, waiting silently.

"I know about the twins' true identities," she said finally. "And the house fire."

She expected Alice to looked shocked or gasp. But the woman kept her green eyes on Sydney, barely moving. She finally took a deep breath and let her shoulders drop.

"I've been carrying that secret for a long time," she said.

Sydney felt the pain and the anger that surrounded Jack's death resurface. "Why didn't Jack tell me about his real name? Or how his parents died?"

"It happened a long time ago," Alice said, looking past Sydney. "When the boys were just teenagers. I worked as a school counselor at their high school in New Hampshire. I had spoken with them on several occasions and knew there was trouble at home. Domestic violence. Verbal abuse. It broke my heart," she said. Sydney could see her eyes become slightly glassy. "So, when they came to me, after the fire, I helped them escape. Start a new life. Finish school. They were finally free of a difficult childhood."

"Jack never told me," she said as the pain burned in her throat.

"I know, Sydney. He wanted to, and he may have one day, if..." She didn't finish the sentence. Sydney didn't need her to, she had been living with what-if's ever since he died. *But he's gone.* She shifted her thoughts back to the more urgent reason for her visit. *Lizzy.*

"So is that what Lizzy found out? That Ethan wasn't who he said he was? And that's why she was murdered?"

The look of shock now registered on Alice's face. Her eyes widened for a moment and then relaxed. "Sydney, I had nothing to do with Lizzy's death, if that's what your implying."

"Well, something happened to her. I know she uncovered whatever was in your secret cabinet. Was it the birth certificates I found?"

Alice took a deep breath and sighed. "There is much more going on here than you realize. Far beyond what happened in the past."

"So tell me, what *is* going on?" she said.

Alice looked at her, fiddling with the sleeve of her bathrobe. "The less you know the better."

Sydney felt a surge of anger flood through her body. She was tired of being a pawn in whatever game was being played here. Half-truths, hidden pasts, and fake identities weren't going to cut it anymore. Her friend was dead and a man just tried to attack her during a couple's massage. She sat up in her chair and slammed her hand on the lacquered wood table.

"Listen, Alice. I am tired of everyone feeding me bullshit answers. Either you tell me what you know, or I'll share my photos of the birth certificates on my Instagram feed."

"You wouldn't do that to Ethan."

Sydney narrowed her eyes at Alice. "Try me," she said.

The two women stared at each other for a moment, seeing who would blink first. Alice had a toughness about her that had intimidated Sydney at first. But after everything she had been through, she refused to let anyone get the best of her. She kept still, staring at Alice, willing her to spill the beans.

"Okay, fine," said Alice, breaking their trance. "You haven't known Jack and Ethan too long, have you?"

"It's been a little over a year." As Sydney said the words, her gaze drifted to the upper right corner of the room, as the memories of Jack tried to pull her into the past.

Jack was one of those people whom she had met at just the right place, in the right time. Two years ago she found herself jaded and alone. Well, not totally alone; both she and Marissa had recently ended relationships. They were back on the singles scene but as a team.

It was a Thursday, or maybe Friday? In those days, all the martini-soaked evenings ran together. This night was somewhat special, as it was her birthday. Sydney was unlucky enough to be born in the dead of winter, just after Christmas in January, when no one had any money left for gifts and the weather in the Midwest was just short of arctic. Not a great time of year for al fresco dining or an outdoor birthday party.

Marissa and Sydney had stashed themselves away in the corner of Mic's Martini Bar & Grill in downtown Chicago. They were drowning their sorrows in dirty martinis and calamari bites but still laughing and having a good time. Just as they were about to head home to sleep off their vodka-sponsored hangover, two fresh glasses arrived.

Smiling from the bar were not one, but two tall, good looking men. Sydney nearly choked on her blue cheese–stuffed olives. She wondered if there was absinthe in her glass, because there was no way identical twins could be that perfect. Both of them had thick brown hair with auburn highlights that caught dim red lights from the bar, and they each stood over six feet tall with broad, muscular shoulders that held lean frames. But even from across the room, she could pick out some distinguishing features. Jack, whose name she would soon learn, had a closely cropped beard and longer hair. He had a more rugged look to him. Ethan, on the other hand, was clean-cut and freshly shaved, and he wore a preppy sport coat. Both men were striking on their own, but standing next to each other, you couldn't help but stare.

She smiled at Jack, and with a slight nod of her head invited him over to join them. The air of charisma around the two men was almost palpable. On that night, as they laughed and got to know each other, she knew that Jack was going to be in her life for a long time, possibly forever.

What she didn't know until now was that he had been lying to her from day one. She shuffled her thoughts back to the present.

"You're a smart woman, Sydney," said Alice. "Do you think it's possible that there were a few things that you didn't know about your husband and his brother? I know that you post a lot of your life on social media, but did you ever wonder why the brothers did not want their pictures taken?"

Sydney wanted to be offended, but Alice had a point. She looked down at her hands. *How well had I known Jack? We'd only been together a year before he died.*

Sydney sighed. "Yes, it's possible." She looked back up at Alice and straightened her shoulders. Jack and Ethan rarely had their photos taken—something about owning a well-known company and keeping their online resume clean. In fact, neither of them had a Facebook page or even a LinkedIn profile. It wasn't completely unheard of for someone in their thirties to opt out of the world of social media, but Sydney did find it odd.

"The truth is that the brothers changed their identities so they could have a fresh start. And they had a good run, while it lasted. But some of Ethan's old habits got them in trouble. He has made some poor decisions that have not only put DoubleDownCasino.com at risk, but possibly even his life at risk."

"Why?"

Alice cocked her head and gave Sydney a thoughtful look. "Did you ever wonder where the boys got the seed money to start DoubleDownCasino.com?"

"Well, Jack told me they took on investors."

"One investor. His name is Vincente Estavez—or the Latin Gangster, as many people in the gambling world refer to him. He was and is a very dangerous man. He found the brothers while he was searching for a partner to start operations in the U.S. The FBI has been trying to bring him down for years, but they can't find a way to break into his inner circle." She brushed a piece of her hair behind her ear and leaned in to the table. "That is, until Ethan and Jack came along."

Sydney stared at Alice in disbelief. She knew that DoubleDownCasino.com had to operate in some legal grey areas to make the business work, but the idea that the investment funds came from a South American gangster seemed like a bit of a stretch. But considering the events of the last forty-eight hours, Sydney was more willing to suspend her disbelief than ever.

Alice leaned back again. "I believe that it was Estavez who had Lizzy killed. He wanted to send a message." Alice paused for a moment, letting the idea hang in the air between them. She reached forward and placed her hand on the gun. "And that is why I have a gun. Because I would do anything for Ethan, but I don't want to die."

Sydney studied her, trying to decide what to believe. She knew Ethan had a habit of getting into trouble; it had only taken a trip or two with him and Jack to Las Vegas before she realized that Ethan had a bit of a gambling problem. But to be involved with someone as shady as Estavez? Not only was he putting himself at risk, but Marissa might be in danger as well.

The pieces of the puzzle started to fall together in her mind. Jack and Ethan's sudden trips to Costa Rica for business. Alice's locked filing cabinet. The FBI's sudden interest in Lizzy's death.

Alex!

Did Alex know about all of this and not tell her?

Of course he did.

Sydney felt anger spread like a heat wave over her body. She had trusted Alex, put her faith in his intentions to help find Lizzy's killer. Maybe even let her guard down. And he had failed to share any of this with her.

Sydney suddenly stood up, causing the gun to wobble on the table. She straightened the front of her dress and began stamping toward the door.

"Thank you, Alice. You've really helped shed some light on this whole thing," she said as she strode past her.

Alice turned her head, watching as she reached the door. "Where are you going?"

"There's someone I need to talk to."

TWENTY-ONE
SYDNEY

AS SOON AS Sydney arrived back in her room, she threw her hat and glasses on the bed, untied the long braid in her hair, and plopped down on the small sofa near the side of the room open to the beach. She tried to take a deep, calming breath, but her body was still rigid with anger after learning the truth. She stood up again and pulled the sliding glass doors open, letting the ocean breeze flood her room with salty air.

It seemed that everyone around her had been lying. Sydney didn't know whether to think she was naïve or just incredibly stupid. She had been *married* to Jack. They had shared a bed, a life, even toothbrushes. How could she have spent so much time physically with someone and not even know his real name? Or where he was from? Their whole marriage had been built on lies. From his past to his involvement with an international criminal.

To Jack, she had been an open book. Ready to share any part of her life she could, willing to be vulnerable in order to bring them closer together. Jack had appeared to reciprocate, sharing his hopes and dreams, but she realized now that he had been tight-lipped about his past.

Damn it! Sydney thought, pounding her fist on the table next to her. It seemed futile to be angry with him. He was gone. But the feeling was still there, even more so since she couldn't ask him why he had decided to conceal the truth.

And then there was Alex. She knew it was dangerous to trust an FBI agent whose only job was to spy on her friends for evidence. But he had won her over, slowly. He had a way with her that made her feel confident in her real self—not just the person she was online—but at the same time, question everything about her life. She wondered if she was attracted to how he made her feel or who he really was.

Even though they had spent the last few days together, she really knew nothing about him. The connection had felt real, but now she was questioning her own intuition. Maybe it was all in her head, just like it had been with Jack. In fact, she wondered if Alex was even his real name. Apparently a real name was optional in the circles she ran in.

She looked up and stared at the TV, which was tuned to the hotel's home channel. A carousel of photos were dancing across the screen showing off the resort's beautiful architecture and lush landscaping. The photos featured happy couples laughing on the beach, having dinner, enjoying a couple's massage. *All lies*, Sydney thought. Just like the picture-perfect life she had led was a lie too.

She knew Alex would be there any moment. While they were on the plane en route to Jamaica, he had typed a cell phone number in her contact list to get a hold of him in case of an emergency. She had sent him an emergency message as she stormed back to their room indicating she needed to speak with him *now*. She continued to pace the room, ready to explode at any moment. Finally, Alex burst through the hotel door.

"Sydney! Are you okay?" he said, his eyes searching her for any sign of harm as the door clicked shut behind him. She turned and glared at him.

"You lied to me," she said as she charged across the room. She stood just a few inches from him and poked her finger in his chest. "You've been lying to me along with everyone else. This isn't about finding Lizzy's killer. You already know who did it!"

Sydney had to fight back tears as she talked. "You're here because you want to bring down Vincente Estavez. Break into his inner circle. Probably trying to win the next FBI trophy or whatever they give you for arresting international criminals. You're just using me to get to him!" She shoved her finger deeper into his chest and then dropped her hand to her side.

"Sydney, slow down. There is more to the story." He reached up and put his hands on her shoulders. She quickly stepped out of his grasp.

"More to the story? My friend is dead! What about her story? What about the family and friends who loved her, the life she still had ahead of her? Maybe to you she was just another byproduct of an ongoing criminal case. But she was *my friend*," she said as she pointed at her own chest.

"Sydney, please listen to me. I know Lizzy was important to you. We want to bring her killer to justice. But it's complicated. There is an international criminal involved. The FBI is barely inside their jurisdiction—one wrong move and we lose control of this case. And that means Lizzy's killer may never be brought to justice."

"Well, let me make things a little less complicated for you. I'm leaving. I refuse to be a part of this anymore. You are on your own." She pushed past Alex and pulled her suitcase out of the closet. She dragged it across the room and threw it on the bed.

"Sydney, wait. Let's talk about this."

She ignored him and continued to stamp around the room, throwing her clothes, toiletries, anything she could find toward the suitcase on the bed. Alex kept his eyes on her, watching calmly. She reached down and picked up a pale peach scarf. It had been a gift from Lizzy after Jack died.

Sydney stood and stared at the scarf in her hands. She began to tremble. The dam of emotions finally broke free, and Sydney started to cry uncontrollably. She had never felt so lonely, defeated, sad, and angry in her life.

Alex stepped forward and reached his arms around her. Despite her best effort to resist, she let him hold her as she cried. She was still angry with Alex, afraid to trust him, but more than anything she just needed a shoulder to cry on. She stood in his arms for a few minutes, letting all the emotion of the last few days run free from her body. Anger, fear, frustration, sadness, guilt came like waves through her tears.

Sydney finally pulled way, wiping away the makeup-filled tears from her eyes. Alex reached over and grabbed the box of tissues sitting on the TV cabinet next to her. He sat down next to her, handing her tissues while she took a few deep breaths.

"I'm truly sorry about Lizzy. And I'm sorry I didn't tell you about Estavez. I had strict orders to keep you in the dark. Trust me, the less you know the better."

Sydney let out a small sigh. "You know you're the second person to tell me that today."

"Really?" he said, looking at her curiously. "Who was the first?"

"Alice. She was the one who told me about Estavez."

"I see. Well, I don't know what she told you, but Estavez is a very dangerous man. He's wanted for a wide range of international crimes but mainly for his online gambling activities, which falls under the jurisdiction of the FBI. Which is why they sent me here with you."

Sydney sniffled and pulled another tissue out of the box. She dabbed her eyes.

"So, do you think he killed Lizzy?"

"It's the best lead we have so far. Though he's never been convicted, Estavez has been connected to several murders that involved poisoning." He shrugged. "It does make sense."

"How does killing someone ever make sense?" Sydney said, fighting back her tears again.

"It doesn't," he said, reaching an arm around her shoulder. "I'm sorry, Sydney."

"Thanks," she said weakly. They sat side-by-side, and she leaned into him for a moment, needing the comfort. "What happened to the man from the massage room? Was he one of Estavez's guys?"

"I think so. Let's just say he's spending the afternoon getting to know some of my colleagues from the FBI."

"Sounds like fun," she said with a note of sarcasm in her voice. "So, what do we do now?"

"Well, we carry on with the original plan. I'll be your date at the rehearsal dinner tonight and for the wedding tomorrow. That will give me a chance to get close enough to Ethan and win his trust. Once I do that, I can see if he's willing to work with us to bring down Estavez." He let his hand drop down to Sydney's back and pulled away to look at her. "But I need you to really sell the idea that I am your date, maybe even your boyfriend, or it won't work."

Sydney groaned. "I know, I know. It's just hard for me; I'm not ready for the scrutiny. Jack's only been gone for six months." She looked up at the TV screen again, which momentarily froze on a beautiful couple taking their wedding vows on the beach. It was as if the hotel was reading her mind.

"It's only for one night. Then you can just tell people it didn't work out, and how that Alex guy was a total jerk."

Sydney smiled giving him a nudge in the ribs. "Well, not a total jerk." Alex smiled in return. Sydney began running scenarios for the evening through her mind. "We need a good backstory. How we met. Any ideas?"

"Hmm. We met a bar? Dollar draft night?"

Sydney nearly laughed out loud. "Um, no. I would not be caught dead in a bar that serves one-dollar drafts." Alex shrugged and leaned back against the foot of the bed, taking his hand away from her back. "Not that there is anything wrong with those kinds of bars—it's just not plausible."

She stared at the sliding glass doors that opened up to the beach. "How about this: we met at a coffee bar while you were in town on business. Our coffees got mixed up, and you ended up with my sugar-free caramel soy latte. We talked, you asked for my number, and I said no. We would have parted ways, but just as I was getting ready to walk out the door, it began to pour down rain. I stepped back inside, and you came to my rescue with a large black umbrella. Ever the true gentlemen, you walked me to my car and gave me a business card. I lost the card, but weeks later, we saw each other again at the same coffee shop, and you ordered me a sugar-free caramel latte, and we sat down and began to talk. The rest is history."

"Wow. You just came up with all that?"

Sydney smiled. "I watch a lot of Netflix."

Alex laughed. "I see. Well, that works for me."

She suddenly stood up, as if a weight had been lifted from her. "Great! Listen, I've got to hop in the shower. We have a rehearsal to get ready for." She quickly grabbed a few toiletry bags from the bed and headed toward the bathroom.

"Sydney."

She turned around to look at him. "Yes?"

"Just so you know, in real life," he said with a half smile on his rugged face, his grey eyes twinkling, "I would have never let you get in that car without getting your number first."

Sydney felt her heart flutter a bit. She didn't say a word, just smiled and walked into the bathroom.

Maybe Alex wouldn't be such a bad date after all.

TWENTY-TWO

ETHAN

DAMN IT, Ethan thought as his phone buzzed again. Marissa was glaring at him as the wind sent her hair swirling in long ribbons around her shoulders. They were standing on a custom-made wooden platform that floated over the white sand beach just twenty feet from the edge of the ocean tide. Overhead he could hear seagulls squawking, circling the large pergola that had just been erected for tomorrow's ceremony. He and Marissa were supposed to be giggling through the rehearsal of their wedding vows, preparing for tomorrow like most couples. Instead Ethan felt tense and distracted. His phone buzzed again.

"Honey," said Marissa, tucking a long strand of hair around her ear. She was glowing in the fading sun, her long white, off-the-shoulder dress nearly iridescent. Her expression wasn't as pleasant. "Do you need to answer that?"

"I'm so sorry," he said to Marissa and then looked at the wedding officiant standing patiently in front of them. He pulled the phone from his pants pocket and looked at the screen. It was Estavez. "I need to take this."

He looked back at Marissa and leaned forward to kiss her. "Can you finish without me, darling?"

"Okay," she said weakly. He knew Marissa was too proud to ask him to do otherwise.

"Thanks," he said and stepped off the platform. As he made his way toward an empty path that led into the jungle of trees, he swiped the screen on his phone.

"Hello?" he said once he was out of earshot.

"Hola, Ethan. How is my business partner today? Ready for the big wedding?" He heard Estavez's voice crackle over the phone.

"Hi Vince. Yes, we are actually going through the rehearsal."

"Oh, I am sorry to bother you, my friend, but I just wanted to make sure our plan is on track?"

"Yes, I will have the money for next week, once everything is official."

"Wonderful, Ethan. I really do like you, mi amigo. I would hate for our relationship to turn sour."

Though Estavez sounded forcefully cheerful over the phone, the undertone was clear: deliver the money you owe me, or else your life is in jeopardy. His partner had no idea how exactly he would extract the money from his new wife. All he knew was that as soon as he was married, the money would follow. Estavez was willing to wait, but not for long. He wasn't the type of person you wanted to keep waiting. Estavez peppered him with a few more questions about some upcoming campaigns they had scheduled for the website before saying goodbye.

As he walked through the dense jungle, Ethan thought back to the night when everything began, five years ago. He had just finished a hard workout at the gym, his cure for a painfully dull day at the office. He had dropped by his apartment, showered, and walked a few blocks down the street to find his usual stool at the bar.

The sales position he'd landed at a large commercial construction company wasn't exactly allowing him to live his dream life. Everything about the company was bland and boring, from the squat concrete buildings to the grey-beige walls in every room. The small cubicle he called home from 8:00 a.m. to 5:00 p.m. quickly turned into a veritable prison, only missing the iron bars.

He was partway into his second glass when he noticed a guy, about his age, sidle up to the bar. The man, whom he would later learn was named Pete, was chatting with the bartender about how much money he was making at his new gig. When Ethan overheard twenty thousand dollars a month, he put down his beer nuts and waited for the right opportunity to invite himself into the conversation.

After buying Pete a few drinks, not only did he find out exactly how he was making that kind of money, he had the name of someone he could reach out to if he was interested. Ethan had everything he needed.

He threw a couple of twenty-dollar bills down on the sticky bar top and headed home. Jack was asleep on the lumpy brown couch when Ethan burst into their apartment.

"I've got the answer to our money problems!" Ethan announced. Jack sleepily opened one eye and glared at him.

"What time is it?" he asked.

"It doesn't matter. You need to hear this," Ethan continued excitedly, relaying the entire conversation he'd had at the bar with Pete. Jack instantly saw the same opportunity.

"And here's the best part," Ethan continued, "this guy Pete was thinking small, running just one affiliate website. What if we created an entire suite of websites that directed traffic to these online casinos? If one site could generate twenty thousand dollars a month in revenue, imagine what five or ten sites could do?" He was nearly breathless as he waited for Jack to agree.

"I love the idea, man, but we've never done anything like that before. How are we going to build a network of websites?"

Ethan looked at his brother, his twin, and with all the intensity he could muster, replied, "Exactly how we've gotten this far, Jack: we figure it out together."

The next morning, he and Jack skipped their respective jobs and spent the entire day in the living room of their seven-hundred-and-fifty-square-foot apartment, hacking away on the keys of their laptops. Hours became days, and by the end of two weeks, they had a collection of fifteen referral sites that drove traffic to various online casinos, including a Costa Rican–based website called Rico-Casino.com.

The business model was fairly simple. They paid for traffic to their collection of websites. A certain percentage of users opted in to their bonus offer, which redirected them to the casino. Once they arrived at the casino's website and entered their credit card information, they were hooked. Not only did the brothers earn a commission for sending the user to the site, they also received a small percentage of whatever the customer spent on the site.

The first few months were a flurry of late nights hunkered down in Ethan's apartment drinking Red Bull until the wee hours of the morning. Food delivery services became the norm, and what they lacked in sleep they made up for with coffee.

Six months later, he and Jack were working in a small office above the bar where he had met Pete. They had five employees all working at folding tables with laptops, modems and monitor wires snaking through the room like small tributaries of money.

Late one afternoon, Ethan received a call from a Costa Rican number. Jack had told him to ignore the call, as they were in the middle of a meeting, but Ethan instinctively answered the phone. To his surprise, the soon-to-be-familiar voice of Vincente Estavez was on the other end.

Estavez was notorious in the online gambling world, a Costa Rican mogul with a reputation as someone you did not want to cross. He ran RicoCasino.com, which was one of the most popular and successful online gambling sites. Ethan was sure it was no coincidence that it was one of the main sites they had been sending traffic to.

Ethan immediately switched to speakerphone for Jack to hear the call.

"Mr. Estavez, I've got my brother, Jack, on the line as well. What can we do for you?"

"Jack, Ethan, please call me Vince. My head of marketing has been telling me wonderful things about you. You've been sending a lot of good traffic to our site."

"It's our pleasure, Vince," Ethan said, not sure where Estavez was going with the conversation.

"Listen, I've got a business proposition for you. I'd like to fly you down to my headquarters in Costa Rica so we can talk in person. Is that something you would be interested in?"

He and Jack exchanged looks.

Ethan quickly responded. "Uh yes, we'd be up for a visit. When were you thinking?"

The next day, the two weary brothers were on an international flight to the South American country's mountains and beaches. They had barely slept that night, making sure that everything they had built up was in order so they could take a few days off without the entire operation collapsing.

A black stretch limo greeted them upon arrival. The chauffeur handed them warm towels with lemon to wipe their travel-worn hands and poured them each a glass of iced champagne. At that moment, Ethan realized that Estavez was grooming them for something big.

As they pulled in front of the five-star resort hotel, their concierge presented them with an itinerary. The meeting they had flown thirty-five hundred miles for, however, had to wait. He and Jack were surprised to see that for the next twenty-four hours, they would be zip-lining in the mountains, dining at a Michelin-rated restaurant, and partying at the top clubs in San Jose. It wasn't until the following day that they had scheduled a face-to-face with the mogul himself.

The next afternoon, their limo driver took them on an hourlong drive into the countryside. They pulled up to a sprawling estate with seven-foot-tall white stucco walls surrounding the property. A large iron gate opened to the sun-bathed property surrounded by rolling hills and punctuated with several tall watchtowers. The towers and the gates had a visible armed presence, with a small army of men holding machine guns close to their chests.

After they had cleared the entrance, they pulled up to a large circular driveway with a twenty-foot-tall fountain in the center. Bare-chested mermaids sprayed water into the blue tiled pools below. A beautiful woman with waist-length glossy black hair and dark brown eyes was waiting next to a staff of people just outside their car. The sharply dressed woman introduced herself as Ester. She escorted them to a large patio, where handwoven rattan fans circulated the island's air throughout the alcoves.

Vincente Estavez rose from his chair to greet them. He was a barrel-chested man who's presence overshadowed the rest of the people in the room. He wore a white linen button-down shirt that set off his tan skin and slick black hair. A cigar dangled from his gold-ringed fingers.

"Ethan, Jack. Welcome to my home," he said as he reached out and shook their hands.

"Thank you for having us, Vince. This place is beautiful."

"Thank you mi amigo. I trust you enjoyed your stay so far?" said Estavez.

Ethan and Jack exchanged grins. "Absolutely, we appreciate the royal treatment," Ethan responded.

Estavez laughed. "Royal treatment—I like that."

He gestured to a uniformed employee near him. A few seconds later, a tray of fruit, pastries, and drinks was placed on the coffee table in front of them. "So let's cut to it. I know you are wondering why you are here."

Ethan fumbled to find the right words. "We are."

"As you can see, business has been good," Estavez said as he gestured to his surroundings. "But, it is becoming more difficult for me to get past all the regulations and bureaucracy that my government—and yours—has created." He paused and waited for the brothers to nod. "Not only that but my business partner and I have not been seeing eye to eye."

Ethan noticed the women who had escorted them into the patio area shift uncomfortably behind him. It was a subtle movement, but Ethan quickly picked up on it.

"I would like to set up a site that has a little more credibility, and I need an American team to do it. This partnership would be extremely lucrative for whomever I choose to work with." He paused for emphasis, taking a long drink from his glass. "That's where you come in. You've showed some promise and ingenuity with your business, and I would like you to launch my new casino."

Ethan looked at Jack again and leaned forward in his chair. "With all due respect, you need more than just an American team, Mr. Estavez; you need American owners. We know the laws. If you want us in on the deal, you have to make sure your name stays off the paperwork."

Ethan's heart was pounding wildly. It was a bold move on his part, but he knew guys like Estavez didn't want to work with cowards.

"I see you are a smart man, Mr. Evans." Estavez paused, talking a draw from his cigar. "But I also know you don't have the connections and the funds to pull this off on your own. I'm willing to offer all of that and more, for a sixty-forty split."

The negotiations went on from there, and when they had finally negotiated a fifty-fifty split, Estavez laid out the rest of his plan to launch their new online empire.

When they returned home, it felt as though their entire life had been upgraded. They leased a large office space with exposed brick walls and a full-service coffee bar. They hired more staff to support their new venture. Double-DownCasino.com was a law-abiding, flourishing start-up as far as anyone knew.

Flush with cash and newfound success, Ethan got a little sloppy. He started renting private jets to fly himself, Jack, and their small group of friends out to Las Vegas for three-day weekends of partying and gambling. Estavez had deep connections within the industry and landed Ethan a seat at some of the most exclusive poker tables in Vegas. That's when Ethan started getting himself into debt with the wrong people.

Of course, Estavez was waiting in the wings, eager to bail Ethan out of trouble. That's when the relationship between the twins and the Costa Rican gangster began to sour. With Ethan's back against the wall, Estavez decided to change the terms of the deal. He wanted to cut the brothers down to only twenty percent of the profits, even though they had done all the work to get the site where it was. Ethan was furious. There were some heated phone conversations among the three of them, but Estavez refused to back down, threatening to throw Ethan to the wolves.

Jack had insisted they fly down to Costa Rica, to work out a deal with Estavez face-to-face. He was furious with Ethan and frustrated at the situation. He'd been a licensed pilot since they graduated college and told Ethan that some time in the sky would clear his head. Ethan was going to meet him there. But Jack didn't make it.

Ethan shivered in spite of the heat, thinking about his brother. He shifted his thoughts back to the present.

He was far away from the ceremony site now, outside the bounds of the resort. He had followed a path that led into a thick bundle of trees and bushes. He retraced his steps and started walking back toward the crowd of people now populating the pool area. The sun was lowering in the sky over the ocean, changing the colors of the waves from turquoise to a murky blue. From a distance, he could just make out the silhouette of his soon-to-be wife.

Or rather, his soon-to-be-*dead* wife.

TWENTY-THREE

ETHAN

"ETHAN, THERE YOU ARE!" Marissa said, charging in his direction. She was slightly breathless when she finally caught up to him.

"I'm sorry, sweetheart. I was caught on a work call," he said, kissing her hand in a gesture of apology. "It won't happen again."

"It better not." Marissa arched a perfectly shaped eyebrow at him. "Now, come on, we have a party to host."

He looked around the rehearsal dinner as she led him to the head table. The palm trees were heavy with crystals and small LED lights that gave the effect of twinkling icicles reflected in the pool. White linen-lined cocktail tables were placed throughout the area and an army of servers were offering drinks to all the guests who had gathered for the evening.

The ebb and flow of laughter revealed a more cheerful mood than the night before. He could see that people were more comfortable moving on from the incident with Lizzy than they were dealing with their grief. Ethan was relieved because he had his own plan to execute, and the incident on the jet had nearly derailed the entire operation.

The plan he had put into place was rather simple. He and Marissa would be wed tomorrow in a highly anticipated ceremony. But it was what would happen after the wedding that would send an unexpected shockwave through the tabloids.

Upon the official signing of the wedding documents, the prenuptial agreement that he and Marissa signed would become legal and binding. In the event of her death, he would not inherit her entire fortune, as some tabloid trash had speculated. Instead, he would receive a large lump sum via a life insurance policy, their home in Chicago, and a generous share of stock in her company. To an outsider, this wouldn't seem important to Ethan because of his own successful business. But because of the debt he owed to Estavez, this money now meant life or death to him.

Given that Marissa's entire fortune was tied up in multiple trusts, with layers upon layers of protection, it would be nearly impossible to extract the money he needed from her while she was alive. Even if she wanted to give him the money, it would be a legal nightmare to do so. That was the catch of extreme wealth—it seemed the more money you had, the less control you had over it.

And so, he'd had a choice to make: his life or Marissa's. And while Marissa was beautiful, rich, and a tomcat in the sack, he wasn't ready to die. Not yet.

As they crossed over a footbridge arching over the glistening pool, he spotted Sydney wearing a deep red dress. She was arm-in-arm with the mystery man from the airport that his PI Bishop had told him about. The sight immediately threw Ethan off balance. He wasn't used to seeing Sydney with anyone other than his dead brother.

"Sydney!" he heard Marissa yelp next to him.

Marissa grabbed his arm and nearly dragged him to where Sydney and her date where standing. As they drew closer, Ethan looked him up and down, taking in his perfectly straight posture, muscular physique, and sharp clothing. Bishop had been right; the guy certainly gave off an ex-military vibe.

The girls exchanged cheek kisses, and complimented each other on how beautiful they looked. Marissa looked at Sydney's date, then smiled slyly at her, seeming happy that her best friend was dating again. Ethan hung back a few steps, observing their exchange. Sydney looked genuinely happy to see Marissa, but when her eyes fell on him, she seemed to clam up.

"Ethan, how are you," she said, leaning in for a quick hug. There was a palpable tension between the two of them.

"I'm good. Glad you made it, Syd," he said, glancing at the man next to her. The way she was standing so near to him displayed a certain level of comfort between them. He looked squarely at Sydney. "I heard you had a bumpy ride on the way here."

"You can say that again!" she said, adding an awkward laugh as if to emphasize her point. She reached over and put a hand on the mystery guest's back.

"This is Alex, my date for the, uh, weekend," she said and added another nervous laugh. "Alex, these are my dear friends, Marissa and Ethan." The way her eyes moved quickly from one face to another gave Ethan the feeling that she was lying about something. What that was, he wasn't sure. But he knew Sydney well enough to know she was a terrible liar.

Alex extended his hand. First to Ethan and then to

Marissa. Ethan noted his firm handshake and the effort to make eye contact.

"Nice to meet you," Alex said confidently.

"Nice to meet you, Alex," he replied smoothly. "Glad you could join us for the celebration."

"Yes, we are so excited that Sydney brought a date!" Marissa blurted out.

Ethan saw Sydney wince as Marissa spoke, then she took a long drink from her cocktail glass. There was a moment of uncomfortable silence between the three of them until a waiter came by with a tray of champagne.

"Excuse me, it looks like it's time for a toast," Ethan said. He grabbed Marissa's hand and headed toward the north end of the pool. He could hear Marissa say something to Sydney as they were leaving, but he was too wrapped up in his own thoughts to hear it. There was something going on with Sydney and her date and he needed more information. His heartbeat began to pick up its pace. If the feds where here, the entire plan he had put together was in jeopardy of falling apart.

He stopped just as they were passing one of the tall cocktail tables and noticed a man in a dark suit was trying to get his attention by jutting his chin at him and raising his eyebrows. He was short with narrow shoulders that hunched forward. He had a plain face with pale features that blended in with the crowd. Ethan wouldn't have even noticed him if he hadn't been intentionally trying to get his attention. It took a few seconds, but then he realized it was his private investigator, Bishop.

They had only actually met in person twice, though he had hired Bishop on and off for the last three years. When Ethan became entangled in the high-stakes poker rooms, he found it useful to know whom he was playing against. The more money Ethan owed to Estavez, the more his paranoia grew. Soon he was having Bishop follow Jack, Sydney, and even Marissa on various occasions, to make sure they weren't lying to him. But despite keeping him employed over the years, he insisted that all their interactions be kept at a distance.

For Bishop to show up like this meant that he had extremely urgent news.

He leaned in and spoke softly into Marissa's ear. "Could you excuse me for a moment, honey? I've got to speak with someone about a little surprise I'm planning for you."

A little flutter of recognition floated across her expression. He wondered if she knew anything about his plan. *You're just being paranoid*, he told himself.

"Of course," she said with a slight smile. "But don't be long." She spotted someone she knew and strolled off in their direction.

Ethan made a beeline for Bishop and stopped just a few feet short of where he was standing. He grabbed another glass of champagne from the nearest tuxedo-clad waiter and motioned for Bishop to join him just outside the lights from the party. When they were far enough away from the guests so no one could hear them, Ethan broke the silence.

"You better have an amazing fucking reason for showing up like this, my friend," he said tersely.

"I do," he said, glancing over Ethan's shoulder. He looked back at him. "I tried texting you, but you didn't answer your phone." Bishop took a deep breath. "I think you are being followed."

"What? By who?" Ethan said. He felt the knots already present in his stomach begin to tighten even more. He wouldn't be surprised if Estavez had someone tailing him, but it still made him uncomfortable.

"I don't know who it is for sure. I arrived at the hotel late this morning and parked my car off the circular driveway to wait for Sydney's transport van. As I sat there, I saw a taxi drive up to the front lobby door and you stepped out. A few minutes later, another taxi arrived and a man stepped out of the car. He seemed to be asking questions to the hotel staff and even slipped them some cash. I found that odd, so I followed him inside."

Ethan felt a chill run up his back. If someone had followed his taxi, they may have seen exactly where he went.

Shit.

"He seemed to be following you, but from a distance. When Marissa arrived, he left, following a group of people out to the pool area. I walked out to the pool, but when I got there, he was gone."

Ethan stared into the darkness behind Bishop, gnawing on the edge of his lip. "Are you sure he was tailing me?"

"I do this for a living, man. I'm sure," he said.

Ethan shook his head. "Okay, thank you for letting me know. Hang around and see if you spot him again. Try to see what he's up to."

Bishop nodded. "Will do."

Ethan walked back toward the party, trying to calm his nerves by convincing himself that it was just one of Estavez's guys and he had everything under control. With Bishop's attention now divided between Sydney, Alex, and this new mystery player, he might need some help.

Ethan could see the twinkling lights up ahead, floating over the crowd of people mingling by the pool. Dusk had settled for the evening, making it difficult to see individual faces. But he knew he could find Sydney and Alex if he kept walking.

If Sydney's date was an FBI agent, Ethan was going to

need to find out why he was there. Estavez would be furious if he knew the FBI was involved, and more than that, it would make Ethan look bad. If Alex did turn out to be FBI, Ethan would likely turn him over to Estavez's men.

If there was one thing Ethan had learned from years of working with the Costa Rican gangster, it was this: he had a way of making people who got in his way disappear.

TWENTY-FOUR

SYDNEY

"YOU DIDN'T ACT suspicious at all," Sydney said sarcastically to Alex, giving him a playful nudge. "Aren't you supposed to be an expert undercover agent?"

She shifted her weight in her nude heels, which were starting to dig into the sides of her feet. The off-the-shoulder red dress she had chosen for the evening just dusted the floor. She'd only had enough time to loosely braid her hair over one shoulder, but it worked with the outfit. She didn't mind the look on Alex's face when she had stepped out of the bathroom. He had told her several times how gorgeous she looked.

Alex stood casually next to her with his wineglass still full of champagne. The way he held his shoulders straight and kept his chin up made him look like a soldier—alert and ready to dive into battle. But his charming smile told another story. When she had leaned in to tease him, she realized he was wearing cologne, a soft oaky smell mixed with his natural scent.

"I wanted to pique his curiosity a bit. Let him know I'm

someone he should watch," he said, taking a small swig of his champagne.

"Why?" Sydney asked, tipping her head to the side.

"Well, part of my assignment is to get him alone so we can have a conversation about the whole situation. But the timing has to be right. If Ethan suspects I'm with law enforcement, he will tread more carefully." His tone had gone quiet. She could tell he was being careful not to speak too loudly so that other guests couldn't eavesdrop on the conversation. "I don't want to make a scene and ring any alarm bells if Estavez has his men around."

Sydney dropped her voice to match the tone of his. "Undercover assignment sounds so James Bond. Are you wearing an earpiece or hiding a small secret camera somewhere?" She gave him an animated once-over as if searching for any clues.

Alex laughed uncomfortably. "No, all I have is my cell phone. No James Bond here."

"Too bad," she said softly, shrugging one shoulder. She sighed. "So what's next? You've met Ethan—what do we do now?"

Alex kept scanning the crowd casually, pretending to sip at his wine. He seemed to be looking back toward a manicured path next to the pool. He responded while barely looking at her. "There may be some other information I can gather just by walking around and talking to guests." He looked back at her and placed a hand on the back of her left elbow as he continued to speak. Despite being quite anxious, Sydney got a small tingle from the gesture.

"I'm going to do a few laps around the crowd, see if I can find out anything useful. Do you think you can handle yourself alone for a while?"

Sydney paused for a beat before giving him an answer.

Truthfully, she didn't want him to stop touching her arm. "Of course, Alex. These are my friends too." And with that Sydney walked off before he could say another word. She sort of hoped he was watching her as she walked away, but more than likely he had refocused on his task.

She was a little disappointed to have to work the crowd on her own. Having someone with her to deflect some of the well-meaning questions from nosy acquaintances had been a nice change of pace. She was dreading seeing old friends, and the all-too-familiar look of pity on their faces. Especially now, after what had happened to Lizzy.

She spent the next forty-five minutes clicking around the delicately lit pool area. She could hear the sound of laughter as guests mingled, and the clink of glasses. Servers were dressed in formal black-and-white attire, floating from one group to the next to keep the hive of energy buzzing and the drinks flowing. She mingled with guests, snapped a few videos to add to the stories section of her feed, and tried to present herself confidently while masking any signs of worry that had her stomach tied in knots.

She spotted a few friends from college—Julie Maxwell and her husband, Daniel—took a deep breath, and headed in their direction. As she approached, she immediately noticed the "look." It was always the same. "Hi Sydney, it's so great to see you." Followed by a head being cocked and a sympathetic "How are you?" She was sure that the concern was genuine most of the time, but it was always awkward.

"Sydney!" said Julie, leaning forward to give her a brief hug. "It's so great to see you. Do you remember my husband, Daniel?"

"Of course," Sydney said. "Great to see you, Daniel." Daniel's attention had left the conversation already. He was studying the rear of one of the waitresses as she chatted with a guest.

Julie and Daniel, like Sydney, had a picture-perfect life on social media. Word had gotten around, though, that Julie's drinking had become a problem in their relationship and Daniel had a wandering eye.

You just never know, thought Sydney. But who was she kidding? Her social media profile certainly didn't reveal the truth about her current state of affairs.

"So, how are you doing? I'm so sorry to hear about Lizzy. I know she was a dear friend of yours," Julie said, giving her a sympathetic head tilt.

"I'm fine," Sydney said, the words catching in her throat. "It's hard, her not being here. But I know she would have wanted to see Marissa and Ethan married." She could feel her cheeks burning as she spoke and was desperate for any opportunity to change the conversation. Julie seemed to pick up on this.

"I see you brought a date! He's cute," she said, giving Sydney a knowing look. "How did you two meet?"

Sydney nearly sighed with relief. This was a question she could handle. "Oh, we just met at a coffee shop in Chicago."

"Well, I'm happy for you, Sydney. It's great to see you out there, dating again, you know since..." She moved her head from side to side, not wanting to call a spade a spade.

"Oh, you mean since my husband died?" She wished people weren't so afraid to just say it.

"Um, yes." Julie took a sip of her drink, clearly embarrassed. Just as Sydney was about to ask some not-so-polite questions about Julie's life, Maxwell appeared next to her. Julie turned her attention toward the butler, obviously looking for a reason to escape the conversation.

"Oh Maxwell, do you need something?" Sydney said.

"Yes, ma'am. But don't let me intrude," he said in his calm, dry manner.

"Oh, it's not a problem," she said as she turned toward Julie and Daniel. "Catch up later?"

"Of course! Enjoy your evening." Julie gave her a tight smile and latched on to Daniel's arm as they walked away.

She turned her attention back to Maxwell. "Is everything all right?" she asked, curious as to why he had found her at the party.

"Yes, ma'am," he said while extending a carefully folded note on his gloved hand. "This note came for you. They said it was urgent."

"Urgent? Who's it fro—"

"I was only asked to pass the note along to you, ma'am. Have a wonderful evening," he said and quickly ducked back into the crowd.

Sydney was still standing there with her mouth open to speak as he disappeared. She looked down at the note in her hand. *What now?* she thought anxiously.

She spotted the nearest vacant cocktail table and squeezed her way through a few couples happily chatting away with drinks in hand. Sydney sat her glass and beaded clutch on the tall white-and-gold-embellished tabletop. The note was folded into a square, and as she unfolded the layers, she found a typed message centered on the page.

Meet me on the beach at 10 p.m. It's urgent.

She stared at the page. There was no signature. *Who is this from?*

She looked around to see if Maxwell was still nearby, but he had gone. She wanted to ask him how he had gotten the note. As she continued to scan the crowd, she saw Alex coming back toward her. She quickly refolded the note and stashed it in her clutch.

She was just putting her champagne glass to her lips as he sidled next to her.

"There you are," he began. "Did I miss anything exciting?"

"Oh no, just catching up with old friends," she said, letting the champagne trickle down her throat. "What about you—any juicy leads you cooked up during your recon mission?"

Alex laughed. "I wouldn't call it a mission. Nothing out of the ordinary actually. Just a bunch of nice people getting sloshed at a rehearsal dinner party."

"Let's join them," Sydney said as she emptied her champagne glass.

TWENTY-FIVE

ETHAN

ETHAN SCANNED the crowd at the rehearsal dinner. Everyone was laughing, and the drinks were flowing. As promised, the wedding planner had delivered an exceptional event that went off without a hitch. Each detail was carefully selected for an elegant beach theme. In a twisted way, Ethan wanted only the best for his soon-to-be short-lived marriage. As he saw the impressed looks on the faces of the guests he had invited, he felt a sense of satisfaction. In a way, he would prove to everyone that he could move on, even from the death of a twin. And he could use their sympathy to his advantage.

Right now, however, he needed to get a location on Sydney and her date, Alex. At the same time, it would look strange if he left Marissa by herself. She was dressed in a long, off-the-shoulder gown that just barely clung to her curves, and he enjoyed the way other men were looking at her. Her long crystal earrings brushed against his nose as he kissed her bare shoulder.

She was doing her best to enjoy the party, although he was sure it was a front. He hadn't seen her without a drink in her hand all night long, and he was starting to worry she might be drinking too much. She was leaning into him as she laughed and chatted with guests.

"Have to get something, sweetie. I'll be right back," he whispered in Marissa's ear.

She turned to him and forced a smile.

"Sure, honey. Don't be long," she said as she kissed him on the cheek.

Ethan pushed through the crowd and made a loop around the pool. It was difficult to move unencumbered as he continued to spot guests who were eager to speak with him. He was careful not to make eye contact as he scanned the lowly lit space for a sign of Sydney.

"Ethan." He heard a familiar voice and stopped. "Great party."

Startled, he turned around and faced the short, wide silhouette of a man wearing a white linen suit and matching fedora. His deeply set hazel eyes and black facial hair gave him an unmistakable look. If there was a style standard for a South American gangster, Vincente Estavez was a trendsetter. The woman standing next to him was his right hand, Ester, whom Ethan had met on his visit to Costa Rica. She was dressed to kill in a plunging silver gown, her long hair snaking over her shoulder. She looked like a South American version of a young Cher, equally as beautiful.

"Vince? What are you doing here?"

"Well, my business partner is getting married tomorrow and I didn't want to miss the big party," he said with a heavy accent.

Ethan felt Estavez sizing him up. He was more than surprised he was at the rehearsal dinner—*shocked* would have been an appropriate word.

Estavez was notorious across the world in online

gambling, but he rarely left Costa Rica. His history was a patchwork of violations, probations, and rumored crimes he snaked his way out of. Monetary success, however, had afforded him the ability to pay off seemingly every cop, government agent, and politician in his home country. He had total safety and security there as long as the money kept rolling in. But outside of Costa Rica, he had little control. So to see him here, in Jamaica, was highly unusual.

Ethan felt his anxiety kick into high gear, sending stabs of adrenaline throughout his body. He gave one last glance in Sydney's direction and then gave his full attention to Estavez.

"You remember my second in command, Ester." She smiled at Ethan as she offered him a long, delicate hand.

"Wonderful to see you again, Ester," said Ethan, recovering from his shock. He stepped back and gestured to both of them with a slight smile. "I'm so glad you are here. I wasn't sure if you would be able to make it on such short notice." He had had Alice send Estavez an invitation just a few days ago, hoping that he wouldn't have time to make arrangements. But he was careful not exclude him from the event, thinking Estavez would find a snub suspicious.

"Would you like to meet the bride?" Ethan said, gesturing in Marissa's direction.

"I would love to," said Estavez, nodding.

"Right this way." He led Estavez and Ester through the crowd toward Marissa, and his heart pounded a little faster in his chest. Ethan knew if he had any future, and wanted to stay alive, he needed to play this situation right. Marissa was just ahead of them, chatting with a couple where he'd left her.

He tapped her delicately on the shoulder.

"Speak of the devil," she said as she turned and gave a wicked smile.

"Who me?" Ethan pointed at himself with an innocent smile. "Marissa, there is someone I would like you to meet. This is Vincente Estavez and his partner, Ester."

Without hesitating, Marissa extended a slender, tan arm out toward her guests.

"Mr. Estavez, Ester: it's so nice to meet you. Thank you so much for coming."

"Señorita, the pleasure is all mine. You are even more beautiful than Ethan has described. Thank you for allowing me to attend your wonderful party."

"It's a pleasure to have you here," she said, keeping a slight smile on her face. Ester stood next to Estavez, perfectly still as they spoke.

Estavez reached down into his pocket. For a brief moment, Ethan panicked, thinking he was going to pull a gun. He took a deep breath to calm himself. Instead, he produced a long white box with a satin bow.

"A gift for the bride and groom."

"Oh, thank you," Marissa said as he handed her the box.

"Please, open it."

"Of course." She handed Ethan her champagne glass, and with one pull the ribbon fell aside. She pulled the top off the box and they peered inside. A long silver knife sat in the box with what looked like an ivory handle. Engraved on the blade was a phrase written in Spanish. Ethan and Marissa looked at Estavez expectantly.

"El amor es ciego pero el matrimonio abre los ojos," he said, smiling slightly. "It's a Costa Rican expression that means 'love is blind, but marriage opens the eyes.'"

For a moment, Ethan thought Marissa was going to drop the box on the floor, knife and all. She quickly recovered.

"Mr. Estavez, this is beautiful. Thank you." Marissa closed the box and put it on the table next to her. "I'll make sure our butler gets it back to our room."

"You're welcome. Now, if you'll excuse me, señorita, I have some business to attend to." He turned to Ethan. "We can talk later."

Ethan watched as Estavez melted back into the crowd, Ester following closely at his elbow.

"He doesn't seem so bad," Marissa said as she playfully nudged him.

Ethan nodded. The message Estavez had just sent was not lost on Ethan. While the knife was expensive and beautiful, it was also *deadly*.

TWENTY-SIX

SYDNEY

"COME ON, let's grab our seats," Sydney said just as dinner was announced by the Jamaican bandleader. Alex extended his arm, and they made their way to their designated table.

She and Alex found their handwritten name cards at a table near the front of the stage and took their seats. Each round table was elegantly covered with a white tablecloth and a pale blue satin table runner. Fresh white lilies, carnations, and roses were artfully arranged down the center of the table in small glass vases wrapped in twine. Bleached sea shells were scattered throughout the space. The rehearsal dinner was more decadent than most of the weddings she had been to, Sydney thought. Marissa and Ethan were just across the pool area at their own private table.

As they dined on striped sea bass, whipped cauliflower, and green beans, Sydney thought about the note. She wondered who it was from. There was only one way to find out. Sneak away from Alex long enough to escape to the beach.

It was an odd feeling to have no one she could really

176

confide in. Although she was beginning to trust Alex, there was still so much at stake. The less he knew about this, the better.

She had barely spoken to Marissa since she arrived, which was for the best because Marissa knew her well enough to know she was hiding something big. She knew she couldn't call her parents—there was no way they would understand and she had enough on her plate right now just trying to sort things out for herself.

Speaking of her plate, she had been picking at her food. She hadn't had an appetite since breakfast, especially with everything that seemed to be happening in high speed. She kept tracking the time on her phone, feeling distracted and anxious.

"Everything okay?" Alex said as he leaned over to her.

"Yes, I'm fine." She sighed, fumbling with the name card on her place setting. "It's just a lot to take in."

"I get it. Listen, you're doing great. The wedding is tomorrow and then this will all be over. You can go back to your normal life."

Sydney sighed and pushed a delicious-looking green bean across her plate.

"I don't know if I want to go back to my normal life. Clearly, burying my head in my social media feed caused me to miss a few things. Maybe it's time for a change."

Alex frowned. "I took a look at your Instagram feed and it was great. You seem to really have a knack for what you do. I wouldn't give it up so soon."

Sydney shrugged. She was touched by his encouragement, but inside she felt conflicted. *Maybe I just need a break*, she thought.

The servers came in and removed their plates, then served coffee and dessert. The smell of warm coffee wafted up to her nose. She sipped and watched Alex chat up the rest of the guests at their table. By the time dessert arrived, he had everyone laughing and smiling while they plunged their forks into the red velvet cake. She noticed Ethan peering over at them from time to time.

When dinner was finally over and a few toasts had been made, they said goodbye to their table mates and began making their way back to their room. Alex kept a careful distance from Marissa and Ethan as he deftly moved through the crowd from one conversation circle to another. Sydney could tell he was keeping an eye on everyone. She moved close to him as he was deep in conversation with a couple from Long Island and whispered, "Ladies room, be right back."

He looked back at her and nodded with a smile. He didn't seem to suspect anything, much to her relief. She wondered if she had built up enough trust with Alex, although in his position, it must be difficult to trust anyone. Knowing that he was most likely keeping close tabs on her, she made a mental note to be careful.

Sydney's heart raced as she casually passed the women's restroom and headed toward the beach. She was to meet her mystery date at 10:00 p.m., and it was about five minutes until then. As she got closer to the ocean, the sound of the waves deepened and the reception music behind her began to fade.

The sun had set hours ago, and there was an almost disturbing quietness that hung in the salty air. She didn't know whom she was looking for and began to feel a bit stupid for coming to the beach alone, considering every-thing that was going on. She decided she would wait until ten minutes after ten before heading back to the party. She was hoping the person with whom she was meeting would spot her first.

As the minutes dragged on, she felt a pang of guilt for leaving Alex back at the party and lying to him about her intentions. She didn't owe him anything, but she found herself liking him more than she should since he wasn't one hundred percent on her side in this whole mess. But if this meeting had something to do with Ethan or Marissa, it was in everyone's best interest she be here.

The breezes coming off the ocean were giving her a chill. It was 10:08. She would wait two minutes more before heading back to the pool area. Just as she was about to turn around and leave, she glimpsed a lone figure about one hundred feet away moving toward her.

Suddenly, Sydney felt a shiver run down her back. *What am I doing?* The note could have been left by anyone, and perhaps that person did not have the best of intentions. As the figure got closer, she started to take a few steps back. The frame looked familiar: broad shoulders, neatly cut linen shirt.

Ethan!

Why would Ethan want to meet with her? Red alarms were going off in Sydney's head left and right. He must have figured out why Alex was here with her. It was hard enough keeping Marissa in the dark; how was she going to convince Ethan that nothing was up?

Before she could second-guess herself, Sydney turned on her heel and began to briskly walk back to the party. Maybe he didn't see her and she could just pretend she didn't see him. It was worth a shot, otherwise things were about to get way more complicated than she could handle.

"Sydney, wait! It's me!"

Without turning around, Sydney froze in the sand. She felt the panic rise in her throat.

Come on Sydney, move! She commanded her muscles to stretch her feet forward but to no avail. She stood where she was, planted like a statue.

As she heard the sound of his breathing get closer, she heard the voice again. "Sydney."

The woodsy, cinnamon smell of his skin hit her first. She already knew who was standing behind her. It took everything she had not to run. Every fiber in her being was screaming danger, but she couldn't force her muscles to move. She felt a ball of adrenaline explode in her stomach, running through her body until her hands shook. When she finally regained control of her leg muscles, she turned around to face him.

Standing before her was not Ethan.

It was *Jack*.

TWENTY-SEVEN

ETHAN

ETHAN SCANNED the party looking for Sydney's petite silhouette. The crowd was winding down for the evening. Many of the white-covered round tables were now peppered with empty seats, the formerly pristine setup now looking slightly disheveled and abandoned. Servers and bussers were moving from table to table, clearing every last fork, knife, and empty glass. There were still couples mingling among the high-top cocktail tables, late night revelers putting the waitstaff to work. Most of the guests, however, had sauntered over to one of the three bars on the property where the party continued on.

Ethan wondered if he would find Sydney there. He hadn't seen her in the crowd for at least the last hour. He saw Alex several times, even caught his eye a few times. The events leading up to dinner had left him feeling anxious.

The presence of Estavez, coupled with Sydney's date and a possible stalker put his entire plan at risk. Everything he had worked to create was meant to unfold quietly; however, now he felt the pressure press down on him. He needed to be in total control for everything to work out the way he wanted, and the unknown guests he hadn't prepared for made him feel like he was losing his grip.

As far as he knew, Estavez had left the party shortly after he presented his gift. Although he'd never been convicted of a crime, it was generally known that he was not a man to be messed with. His rumored behavior included many mysterious deaths, several of which involved a signature stabbing with a knife. Which is why the threat to Marissa was very clear to Ethan.

He finally spotted Sydney heading toward the bathroom area. She was alone. There was something about the way she walked that caught his attention. She seemed to be moving briskly, as if she was trying to sneak away. *Maybe I'm overreacting*, he thought as he headed in her direction.

"Ready to get out of here?" He heard Marissa's voice in his ear as she ran her hand up and down his arm. He could smell the alcohol on her breath.

ETHAN PAUSED. He knew by her tone and the number of drinks his fiancée had consumed that a trip back to the bedroom meant very good things for him. But his head just wasn't in it tonight. All he could picture was Estavez, the knife, and Sydney's stiff date.

"I would love to, babe. But why don't we wait until tomorrow night? Create a little anticipation for our honeymoon? Like we talked about?"

Marissa pouted for a moment, as if trying to decide whether to increase the stakes of her offer or move on. She chose the latter.

"Well, if you say so honey. I will see you tomorrow then." She gave him a sultry kiss on the mouth and headed toward their suite.

"Marissa, wait." He caught her arm as she was walking away. "Make sure our butler escorts you to the room. I don't want anything happening right before the wedding."

She looked at him incredulously.

"Why would something happen to me?" she said, cocking her head. Her words had started to slur together.

He laughed awkwardly. "Oh, I'm probably just being paranoid. You know, with what happened on the jet. I can't bear the thought of something happening to you."

"Oh Ethan, you're so sweet. I see Marcus right over there." She waved to a tuxedo-clad man hanging by one of the hotel buildings. "I'll make sure he gets me to the suite."

She made an about-face and walked in their friend Marcus's direction.

Ethan sighed. They had already agreed to stay in separate rooms that night in anticipation of the wedding. Which was Ethan's idea. He pretended it was a romantic gesture toward his bride, but in truth, he needed time to make sure everything in his plan was ready to execute.

When he saw that Marissa was safely on her way, he turned back to where he had seen Sydney. She was gone.

Deflated, Ethan decided to head toward the beach. Maybe a walk would help him clear his head. He slowly made his way in that direction. He stopped at the edge of the pool and had a waiter bring him another scotch. Drink in hand, he could hear the ocean waves calling to him. The moon was just barely visible through the clouds that striped the evening sky. A storm rumbled far off in the distance; he could feel the air bloated with the impending rain.

As he reached the edge of the beach, he leaned down and pulled his leather sandals off. The sand welcomed his feet, easing some of the tension he felt throughout his body. He arrived at the edge of the water, the sound of the waves crashing louder and louder. He could taste the salt on his lips, mixed with the amber liquid from his glass.

He couldn't see into the dark ocean, but he was sure there were sharks in the water. Waiting for their prey to make the wrong move so they could swallow it up. Although Ethan had always thought of himself as more of a predator than prey, in this moment, he felt like the helpless fish in the water. And Estavez was the shark, waiting and waiting for him to make the wrong move.

He felt trapped. Estavez was well connected. Money had afforded the South American gangster a worldwide reach. And he knew a different kind of people than your average everyday neighbors next door mowing their grass on Sundays. The types of people that knew killers. If Ethan ran, he would be found anywhere he went, on U.S. soil or abroad.

He owed Estavez one million five hundred and forty thousand dollars. It wasn't a small sum for anyone, no matter how wealthy you were. And Ethan's wealth was a front; he didn't have the kind of tangible assets that someone like Marissa had. Everything he had was wrapped up in the website. And truthfully the website wasn't even his since Estavez owned a huge chunk of that too.

He stood facing the ocean and sipped his scotch. The wind ruffled his clothes, sending a chill up his back. Maybe if he stood here all night, he could think his way out of this mess. He looked down at his glass.

"I wish you were here, Jack," he murmured under his breath. The thought brought with it a surge of sadness that bubbled up in his throat. He and Jack would have found a way out, like they always did. Like they did with their parents, together.

But Jack was gone. Ethan had come up with a plan on

his own. One that involved killing his own wife. It was fairly simple. After they wrapped up the wedding reception, Ethan had planned on surprising Marissa with a weeklong trip around the Caribbean in a gorgeous seventy-foot yacht he had rented just for them.

Other than the small staff, they would be alone in the vast blue ocean for days on end to enjoy their newly wedded bliss. He planned to add a heavy dose of Rohypnol to her after-dinner drink during the second night of their excursion. A few sips later, she would become drowsy and pass out. By that time, the boat would be cloaked in darkness. He would slip her body over the side of the boat, and she would drift to the bottom of the sea.

He thought it was a wonderful way to die. One moment you are having the best week of your life, and the next you are just gone. He hoped he would be so lucky one day. From what he knew of Estavez, if Ethan were ever to cross him and get caught, he would not be treated to the same painless demise.

He thought getting the Rohypnol undetected was going to be the most difficult part of his plan. Carrying it on him through the airport felt too risky, so he decided to purchase the drug after they arrived in Jamaica. He'd found a dealer rather easily on the dark web, set up a time to meet, and made the exchange. While Marissa thought he'd been out shopping, he'd actually made a trip to a town called Shettle Wood to complete his purchase. He'd believed his plan had gone smoothly until Bishop had informed him he had been followed.

Ethan looked up the beach to his left. He could see a couple far down the beach, sitting in the sand. He needed to stretch his legs a bit more and headed in their direction.

But just as he started to make out the details of their

silhouettes, he heard a voice call to him from back down the beach, closer to the resort.

"Ethan, wait up!" He stopped and turned. As the man drew closer, he could see it was Alex, Sydney's date for the wedding. *Perfect timing*, he thought as he walked to meet him.

It was time to circle his own prey.

TWENTY-EIGHT

SYDNEY

SYDNEY FELT like her body was on fire and ice cold all at the same time. Her vocal cords were frozen from the moment she saw him. The ocean seemed to grow louder as if to compete with all the voices that were screaming in her head. She found herself holding her breath in one moment and breathing quick shallow breaths the next. Whether it was a panic attack or a heart attack, she imagined they felt the same. *Jack was alive?*

For months after the plane crash, Sydney had waited for news. She had tried to book a flight down to the location near where he landed, but friends and family members had told her to stay and wait. So she waited. And waited. Until she felt so frustrated and sick, she thought she would scream if she didn't do something.

She reached out to Ethan many times during the aftermath of the crash, but he never answered her calls. Marissa later told her that it was too painful for him to talk about. He had accepted that Jack was gone. While Marissa couldn't understand his acceptance, Sydney was too absorbed in her own feelings about Jack's disappearance to think about his reaction. Now she thought maybe Ethan knew he was alive all along.

Jack was a seasoned pilot. As an identical twin, he once explained to her, it was tough to have your own identity. Flying was a way for him to carve out his own niche in the world. He spent hours practicing on the flight simulator. When the weather allowed, he spent almost every Saturday morning up in the sky, logging hour after hour. It had never really bothered Sydney because he was such a capable pilot. He really seemed to take his flying seriously.

That, among other reasons, was why Sydney had not accepted that her husband was gone. She finally broke free of the people trying to support her and flew down to Venice, Louisiana, the nearest Coast Guard station, and demanded answers. What she discovered was deeply disappointing.

The Coast Guard team had retrieved pieces of the plane, luggage, and many of Jack's personal items. There were shredded shirts, torn shorts, and even a shoe he was wearing the day he left. They found the headset she had purchased for him as a Christmas gift. But the last straw was his bracelet. He and Ethan had matching silver bracelets they had worn every day since she had known him. They never took them off. Jack had never really told her the whole story, but she knew it had been a gift from their parents.

When the Coast Guard officer handed her a broken piece of his bracelet, she knew it was over. Jack was gone. Heavy with the news, she rented a car and drove back to Chicago from Louisiana. She spent hours driving the car in silence. Reliving the memories of the last few days they had spent together before he left. Her heart was broken. She also thought of Ethan. His twin. She wondered how he would move on with his life as well. They had spent practically every moment of their lives together since birth. This would crush him.

The day she handed Ethan the broken bracelet was one of the most painful moments in her life. Ethan had said nothing when she handed the bracelet to him; his face was frozen in a stoic expression. Sydney had cried alone in her car for almost an hour afterward.

If that day qualified as her most painful, surely this moment, this day would easily win as the most shocking.

"Sydney. My beautiful Sydney, I've missed you so much." Jack reached out to touch her arm, but she instinctively pulled away. "I have so much to tell you, so much to explain."

It took Sydney a moment before she could form the right words. It was Jack, it was definitely him. His chocolate-brown eyes, wavy auburn hair, and chiseled features were unmistakable. But there was something different. He was thinner, haggard-looking. There was a cold desperation in his eyes that hadn't been there before. Whatever had happened to him in the last six months had changed him.

After she stared at him for few moments, Sydney again found her voice and her words.

"Fuck you."

She turned from him and began to run as fast as she could down the beach.

TWENTY-NINE

SYDNEY

"SYDNEY, wait! Please! Just hear me out."

Jack might have dropped a little weight, but he could still easily outrun Sydney. She slowed her stride and finally came to a stop. They could hear thunder far off in the distance over the ocean. It looked as though a tropical storm was brewing. The clouds shrouded the moon above them, casting an eerie darkness on the beach. Sydney could barely make out Jack's face. They were both breathing heavily. If it wasn't for his unmistakable eyes and his breath so close to her body, she wouldn't have believed he was real.

She finally turned to face him once again.

"What are you doing here? Why are you...why are you alive? You, you lied to me. I thought you were dead! Dead!" She felt the words ring out of her mouth as another wave crashed at their feet. The anger had hit her. She wanted to punch him in the face. Instead, she let out a huffing sound and shoved him.

Jack took a step back and steadied himself.

"Sydney, I know. It doesn't make sense. But I am here

and I want to tell you what happened. If you'll just listen. Please. Let's sit down."

Sydney was so charged with adrenaline that she didn't know if she could sit down. Not to mention the red dress she was wearing was worth about fifteen hundred dollars. But after a deep breath, she sat herself down in the sand and crossed her legs. Jack sat down next to her.

"Okay. I will at least listen to what you have to say. At least tell me why you pretended you were dead. Why you would lie to me like that."

Jack ran his hands through his hair, which he had grown out almost to shoulder length. His beard, though it had been trimmed, was the longest she had ever seen it.

"As you know, I was on my way to Costa Rica to meet Vincente Estavez. Ethan was going to join me in a few days, but he was so keyed up about the whole thing, I thought it would be better to meet with him first, you know, as the voice of reason. I know I told you we had investors when we started DoubleDownCasino.com. The truth is we had one investor: Estavez." Jack looked out over the ocean as he spoke. "He gave us the money we needed to start the company. It felt like a good match. He needed American owners to get past regulations. We got an opportunity to make the kind of money we always dreamed of." He sighed as he stroked his beard. "The problem was that we got into some trouble with the money, or at least Ethan did."

He paused and grabbed a handful of sand and let it fall through his fingers.

"Ethan had started playing some high-stakes tables at the casinos. He went on a few benders and lost some money. Hell, it was a lot of money. To make matters worse, he was trying to invest some of our profits into other start-ups. Insurance money as he called it. When it came time to pay

Vince his share, we didn't have the money. Vince worked with us the first few times, but that only made things worse." He looked down at the sand, shaking his head. "I couldn't control Ethan. He had gotten out of hand."

He stared off into the ocean as if trying to understand his brother. Sydney was sitting there staring at the ocean too. She was too afraid to look at Jack, too afraid to believe he was real. Too angry at the sight of him as well.

"Okay, so why didn't you tell me? Why didn't you tell me you were in trouble before you left?"

"I couldn't, Sydney. I didn't want to involve you. I didn't want you in danger."

"So, what, you left me in the dark? And then you faked your death? Bullshit." She threw a handful of sand in front of her.

"I didn't fake my death. I just..."

"You just, what? Casually forgot to mention you survived? And you've just been hiding out ever since? I deserve an explanation, Jack." She could hear her own voice shaking.

"No, it wasn't like that. The plane hit some weather. It was bad. I wasn't sure if I was going to live through the crash." He paused, looking out over the rolling waves. Sydney felt another chill run across her shoulders. In her mind, the Jack she knew hadn't lived.

Jack continued, "When I hit the storm, it knocked out the navigation system, and I was completely off course. Then, to make matters worse, something lodged itself in the plane's right engine and took it out completely. I had just enough time to grab a life vest and the inflatable boat bag before the plane crashed into the water." His voice quivered a bit as he spoke, as if he were reliving the crash.

Although Sydney was so incredibly furious with Jack,

she empathized with him in that moment. *That must have been frightening*, she thought.

"After I hit the water, I realized I still had the bag and my vest. I was alive. I inflated the boat and floated for a few hours in the dark. That's when I realized I had forgotten to grab my personal locator beacon. I was floating alone in the dark and there was no way for anyone to find me." She could see his hands shaking. "There were sharks in the water. They circled my boat, bumping against the side, trying to knock me out. It was terrifying."

He paused and poured sand over his feet. It was shocking how easy it was to listen to his voice after all this time. The comfortableness of their relationship was still buried in between them somewhere. Even if all the trust was gone.

"A day later I saw a large fishing boat off in the distance. I was able to paddle close enough for them to spot me. They rescued me, fed me. But the time at sea had given me time to think. I came up with a plan that I promised I would follow through with if I survived. So when they picked me up, I made a choice." His voice sounded deeper, more assured. "I didn't know if I was going to regret it later. But I decided not to reveal my identity. I thought maybe if I had some time to think about what to do next, I could get Ethan and myself out of the mess we were in." He turned to look at her. "And keep you out of that mess."

She shot him a dirty look. "I didn't want to be protected. We took a vow. I wanted to be a part of your life. All of it."

"Sydney, I know. I'm sorry. You don't know how sorry I am. But Vince is a very dangerous man. He's killed people. Tortured people. I didn't know it when we first met him. And Ethan wasn't afraid of anything. He wasn't...careful."

"I think he killed Lizzy."

Jack nodded, and looked down at his feet. "I heard about her death. I'm so sorry, Sydney." He reached out his hand as if he was going to touch her shoulder and then dropped it.

Sydney's eyes burned, but she fought back the tears. She refused to let him see her cry.

"Speaking of Ethan, does he know? Did he know this whole time?" She felt a new wave of anger hit her as she waited for his answer.

"No, he doesn't know," he said, looking down at his hands. "Yet."

She turned to face him. "How could you do this to me? To Ethan? Don't you realize how cruel it was? And for what! What was the point of all this, Jack? You just decided not to come back and that was that? Start a new life without us?"

"I did it to save you. Save all of you. Listen, please. I have a plan."

THIRTY

ETHAN

"HEY MAN, can I buy you another drink? We need to talk," Alex said to Ethan a few feet in front of him. The wind had begun to pick up on the beach, causing the palm trees to whip around the resort behind them. He could see that the lights from a few of the outdoor bars were still on. The shadows of customers moved about as they enjoyed late-night drinks.

He sized Alex up for a moment. He was built like a line-backer, with broad shoulders and enough height to match his own. Ethan didn't know if he could take him in a physical fight, especially with the likelihood that he was ex-military.

Hopefully it won't come to that, he thought. He cleared his throat and after a few moments answered, "Yeah, sure. Let's hit the bar."

They walked next to each other silently and stopped at the first outdoor beach bar. It was surprisingly busy at this time of night. People from the reception were coupled up at some small round tables that were flanked by plush rattan chairs. Other guests from the hotel seemed to be enjoying a rowdy nightcap as well. Ethan had always enjoyed the energy of having people around. He was always in his element when he arrived at a bar.

Tonight was a bit different. The pressure he was feeling caused the muscles between his shoulder blades to ball up in knots. Even after a few drinks, he still couldn't seem to relax. It was all he could do to keep up a front for Alex, trying to appear as if he were relaxed and at ease.

They sat down at the corner of the lacquered teak bar and signaled the bartender. The area was a little quieter and private, away from the louder groups of guests.

"So what did you need to talk to me about, man? Sydney's a great girl, if that's what you're asking," Ethan said as their drinks arrived. The words felt bitter on his lips. *Sydney is Jack's girl*, he couldn't help but think. He watched Alex take a swig of his Red Stripe.

"I'll cut right to it," he said. He put his beer down and squared his shoulders with Ethan's. "I know about Estavez. Your connection with him, the business dealings. And I know about your gambling debt. I want to help."

Ethan stared at him, blinking for a moment to let the words register. "I don't know who you are, but this has nothing to do with you, man. And I don't need any more trouble." He began to stand up. "Listen, I have to go." He nodded to the bartender to bring his tab.

"Ethan, wait. I think you'll want to listen to what I have to say."

"Why is that?" He peered down at him in the hazy light.

"I'm with the FBI."

Ethan sat back down at the bar. So Bishop had been right. *Shit*. There was no turning back now; he might as well hear him out. He just hoped that Estavez's men weren't watching him as they spoke.

"FBI? What does the FBI want with me?" he asked, feigning innocence.

"We don't want you, Ethan. We want Estavez. We know you have been working with him under the table. And from what my sources tell me, your business dealings may have taken a turn for the worse."

"My business is completely legit. I have all the legal paperwork to prove it. I'd be happy to have my secretary send you all of our contracts." He paused to take a drink. "I don't think you'll find anything connecting us to Vincente Estavez."

Alex rubbed the bottle he was holding on the bar counter. "I'm sure your paperwork is clean, Ethan. But we have other proof that you are exchanging funds. The bank wires are all traceable. And the sums coincide with your books."

Ethan tensed. "How did you get access to my books?"

"The how is not important," Alex said as he took another drink. "The point is that the Department of Justice has enough evidence to lock you up on pretty serious money-laundering charges for a very long time. I know you don't want to go to jail, Ethan. And we're talking maximum security prison. It's not the kind of place clean-cut guys like you survive very long."

Ethan stared across the bar at the couple on the other end. Their relaxed body language and frequent laughter was a sharp contrast to the panic he felt rising from his stomach. He didn't know if he should punch Alex in the face and run, or sit there and hear him out. He chose the latter.

He turned his attention back to Alex. "Okay, I'll play ball. Even if that were true—and I'm not admitting to anything— what would the FBI want me to do?" He jiggled his glass and nodded to the bartender to bring him another. "Estavez is a smart guy. It'd be tough to pin him down. Even with my help."

Alex took a long pull of his beer. "Pinning him down is our problem. All you need to worry about is saving your own skin. I don't need to repeat the evidence we already have on you."

Ethan knew he was right. He was being hemmed in on all sides. Pressure from Estavez to pay back the debts he owed. Pressure to follow through with his plan. And now he was being pressured by the feds. His brain couldn't work fast enough to process what to do.

"Okay"—Ethan took a deep breath and then a sip of his scotch—"tell me what you had in mind."

Alex looked around the bar as if he was checking to see if they were being watched. He leaned toward Ethan and lowered his voice. "We want to you to get a confession from Estavez." He paused and peered around the room. He then looked back at Ethan. "For killing Lizzy."

Ethan felt as if someone had punched him in the gut. It took everything in him not to shout the next words. "You think he killed Lizzy?"

"I know he did it, Ethan. We have evidence that ties him to the crime scene. Men that have worked for him in the past who were prepping the jet for departure. Partial fingerprints of his cronies on the champagne bottle." Alex looked down at his beer bottle. "But it's all circumstantial. If we can get him to confess, however, we've got a chance to finally capture him and put him away for good."

Ethan stared at Alex in shock. Everything else in the room faded to white noise.

"Why would he confess a murder to me?" he said. It seemed far-fetched that someone as smart and careful as

Estavez would go around bragging about murder. Even if he believed he was untouchable.

Alex looked directly into his eyes. "Because we believe Estavez killed her as a warning to you."

Shit.

Ethan's eyes widened as he leaned back in his chair and looked around the room. The idea that Estavez had killed Lizzy as a warning had been hanging around in the back of his mind, but he had refused to acknowledge it. He scanned the room again, even more paranoid now that someone might be watching them. He had been so preoccupied with his own plan to get rid of Marissa and make a grab for her money, he'd missed making the connection between the two. Fear gripped his chest as he thought about the way Estavez had disposed of Lizzy and then handed his fiancée a knife as a wedding gift. He suddenly got the feeling that even if he paid Estavez off, he was dead anyway.

He tried to think quickly. If he worked with the feds and Estavez found out, he was dead. While he was sure the government could provide him protection for a time, it wouldn't be long before someone slipped up and Estavez found him out. He wasn't the type of person to give up until you were dead. Unless they actually pulled off locking him away in prison.

In that case, he wouldn't have to kill Marissa, leaving him with a lucrative business and a rich wife. Not a bad deal if he could pull it off.

Either way, it seemed that Estavez wanted him dead. Whether he paid his debts or not. Ethan straightened in his bar stool and brushed a hand through his hair. He focused closely on Alex. "Okay, I'm in. On one condition."

Alex leaned back and cocked his head. "And what is that?"

"You can have Estavez, but I keep DoubleDownCasino.-com. Free and clear."

Alex took a drink of his beer and sighed. "You have a deal."

He and Alex made plans to meet first thing in the morning, at a rock outcropping just down the beach from the hotel. A private area where they wouldn't be noticed. Ethan would be wired up just before the ceremony, so the first chance he got to speak with Estavez, he'd be ready.

Once everything had been agreed to, Ethan signed the tab and stumbled back to his room. He barely stopped to take his clothes off before crashing into the giant wooden four-poster bed.

He'd lost count of how many scotches he'd drunk that evening. And although he should have been keyed up and sleepless, anticipating the events of tomorrow, the alcohol had gone to work, numbing his nervous system.

A funny thought hit him that put a smile on his face just before he fell into a deep sleep.

Maybe you could have your wedding cake, and eat it too.

THIRTY-ONE

SYDNEY

"JACK. I've already been a part of your plans. I had plans too. Mine were thrown out the window when you didn't come back. How can you expect me to trust you again?"

Sydney fumbled with the red ruffles on her dress, spreading them out over the sand. She normally would have been more careful not to ruin a beautiful couture dress. But the anger she had boiling in her stomach at this moment was all consuming. The wind swirled around the two of them, pushing her long blond braid over her shoulder.

"Sydney. I still love you." He reached over and took her hand. "You're still my wife."

Sydney snapped her hand away from him as if he stung her.

"Still your wife? Your wife? I don't even know if our marriage was legal. Evans isn't even your real last name!"

Jack stared at her, stunned. "How do you know that?"

"I found the paperwork Alice had been hiding. She told me everything."

She could see Jack's face fall. Clearly her learning about his past hadn't been part of his carefully laid plans.

"I can explain that, Sydney. There are some things in my past. Painful things that I wanted to get away from. Ethan and I, we changed our names legally a long time ago. It was just easier that way."

"You mean things like the fire? Your parents? Why didn't you tell me about all of that?"

She saw Jack's face become flushed and red. He looked away from her.

"I was planning on telling you everything," he said, and he stared off wistfully toward the ocean waves.

"There you go again, talking about plans. I have plans too Jack." She pulled herself up and out of the sand. Her dress whipped around her as she stood, sending a spray of sand across the beach. She shook the sand off her hands.

"I came here with a date. I am moving on with my life. No more lies."

Jack stood up next to her. He brushed away the sand clinging to his arms and legs. "No more lies?" he said. His voice sounded strained, angry. He ran a hand through his hair that was now being blown around his face by the wind. He squinted his eyes at her.

"I am not the only one that lies about their life, Sydney. Do you think that perfect life you portray on Instagram every day is really you? I know it's not, but what about all those people that follow you? The stay-at-home moms and frumpy single women who nearly worship you? Do you think you are being honest with them?"

Sydney stared at him, stunned. She felt her skin bristle with anger. She tried to coil her hair around her hand as her extensions caught in the wind. His words burned through her. Partly because he had no right to judge her and partly because a piece of it rang true.

He continued, "What about when I died? You just

carried on as if nothing happened, nothing to memorialize me or mention my death. It was just back to your picture-perfect life."

"What was I supposed to do? I didn't know how to handle your death! I certainly didn't want to get into a conversation about it with a bunch of strangers on social media!"

"It would have been an opportunity to be real. Maybe actually show them the real side of you, instead of lying to them and making them believe everything was fine."

Sydney was stunned at Jack's words. He had always been so supportive of her career while they were together. Was this what he had really thought all along?

"I inspire women. I wouldn't call it lying, and I would never compare my business to burning down your childhood home and then changing your name to hide it."

Jack took a step back. Sydney had hurt him, she knew it. Maybe she had gone too far.

"It doesn't matter now anyway. I've got my own life to worry about now. You've broken my trust, and it can never be unbroken." She pulled up the edges of her long dress. "Good bye, Jack."

She had been standing in the sand so long, her feet had buried themselves. She nearly stumbled as she started walking back to the hotel behind her.

"Sydney," Jack said to her back as she walked away. "Sydney, wait." He reached forward and grabbed her arm. She was nearly ready to burst into tears and she didn't want him to see her like that: vulnerable. Hurt.

"Just promise me one thing."

"What?" she said, her voice trembling. He had a hold of her arm, but she couldn't bear to look back at him.

"Don't tell Ethan about me. Not yet."

Sydney pulled her arm from his grasp. Without another word she stamped back to the hotel.

By the time Sydney reached the door of her room, she was sobbing. The tears mixed with the layers of makeup she had applied earlier made her eyes sting. She could barely see the silver door handle in front of her. It was all she could do to take a breath and try to calm herself before facing Alex. How would she explain all of this to him? She couldn't. And yet she wanted to, she needed someone to confide in.

When she finally fumbled the door open, she took in the room and saw that it was empty.

"Alex," she called out. The shaky sound of his name betrayed her fragile state. "Are you here?"

She was greeted with silence. Sydney took another deep breath. *What a relief.* The quiet room gave her time to figure out her next steps. If she could even think that clearly.

All the information she had just received from Jack was screeching through her head at a breakneck pace. It was all she could do to keep up with the synapses that must have been exploding with the news. Jack was alive. He had survived the crash. He had lied to her over and over again about everything in his life. *How did I miss this?*

But then, she knew how she missed it. On the surface, Jack fit the bill of goods she was looking for. Charming, successful, handsome, and the list went on. She spent so much of her life portraying perfection that she had lost sight of the depth that lies underneath the surface. There was much more to life than that image she portrayed on social media.

Sydney really thought about what he had said, that she lied. Maybe it was the truth. Sydney only bothered to put out perfection in her feed. She always wore makeup, always had the perfectly styled outfit. She was always doing something *fun.* It was never about the pain she experienced in her life. Her struggles with insecurity. Even the death of her husband, which she dedicated one post to and moved on.

The line between who she really was and the business of being @SydneyStyle11 had blurred. She always portrayed a perfect life because that was the life she wanted to be living. Sydney would often scroll back through her feed each day and admire her work. She wasn't just curating a perfect social media feed; she was creating the perfect life.

Her followers admired it too. As Jack had said, they nearly worshipped her. "How do you keep it together?" they would say. "You are so adorable!" It was constant positive feedback for her, and she was addicted to the feeling it gave her.

But to compare her social feed to Jack's lies? His fake death? *That is ridiculous!* she thought. Her life was unraveling quickly, and she only had a few threads she was holding on to in the first place. When she pulled her hands away from her face, they were covered in smeared foundation and mascara.

Sydney got up off the bed and headed to the bathroom. She wasn't going to solve any problems with all that makeup running in her eyes. She quickly washed her face and dabbed it with a towel. When she looked up at the mirror, she saw the true Sydney, puffy from crying, but truly her. She looked at her reflection for several moments and wondered about her next move. It was late. She was beyond the point of being exhausted and yet she didn't know if she could sleep.

She was shaking as she slipped out of the red dress and into a silk nightgown. Her mind was in shock over the revelation that Jack was still alive. She felt the tears starting to come again.

Just as she was preparing to fall back into her bed, she heard a knock at the door. *Alex?* She thought. No, he had a key.

She grabbed the floral silk robe from the edge of the bed and wrapped it around her as she approached the door. She peered through the peephole. It was Jack.

"I don't want to talk to you anymore," she said through the door.

"Sydney, listen, there is something else I need to tell you."

"Nothing you can say matters now."

"This does. Please, just trust me."

Sydney bit her lip, trying to decide what to do. If Alex found Jack here, she wasn't sure what would happen, how she would explain everything to him.

She sighed and opened the door for Jack. "You need to be quick—my date is going to be back any minute and if he finds you here…"

As she turned to walk into the room, she felt a warm cloth wrap around her nose and mouth, a strong pungent odor stinging her nostrils. She immediately reached her hand up to pry it away so she could catch her breath. But Jack overpowered her, wrapping his arms tightly around her as she struggled.

"I'm sorry, Sydney," he whispered in her ear as she fought to keep her eyes open. "I just can't afford to let you ruin my plan."

Plan. The last word rang in her ears as she finally gave in to the black wave of unconsciousness.

THIRTY-TWO

ETHAN

WHEN ETHAN AWOKE, there was a dry, calloused hand covering his mouth. He pulled back violently as his eyes adjusted to the dim light in the room. Every muscle fiber in his body tightened, his adrenaline sending warning flags to the network of nerves under his skin.

"What the—" He tried to speak, but the words were muffled.

As his eyes adjusted to the light, he saw the man standing over him was his mirror in every way: height, facial features, hair and eye color. Ethan's eyes went from tiny slits to wide open.

No fucking way, he thought. *Jack?*

As his brain tried to recalibrate, he briefly wondered if he had been drugged. But if he was drugged or dreaming, this wasn't the Jack he would have seen. His brother, who now seemed to be standing in his hotel suite, looked different. Thinner, with a slight hollow to his brown eyes. Because of this altered appearance, he was sure what he saw in front of him was real. More than that, he felt it in a way that only a twin could. The shock reverberated through his entire body and made his stomach tighten in pain.

"Ethan, shh, it's me," Jack said.

"Jack? Jack! What are you—why are you...I thought you were dead, damn it!" He fought to break free of Jack's hold on him. Jack took a step back and released his hands from Ethan's mouth. He slowly raised his arms in the air, his body tightly wound and ready to spring away at any moment.

"I know, it's a long story. I'm sorry," he said in a forceful whisper. He raised his hands in front of him, waving them slightly as if to signal surrender.

Ethan was seriously considering knocking his teeth right out of his mouth. The anger hit him like a train, crashing through his sleepy brain.

Jack continued to speak: "Listen, I can explain—"

"You can explain!?" He suddenly felt awake as the news sunk in. "Jack, you piece of shit. I held a funeral for you! How could you do that to me?" He reached out and slapped down one of Jack's hands. Jack stood a little straighter as if knowing Ethan wouldn't kill him right then and there. As he took a deep breath, he concentrated on Ethan's face.

"I didn't plan for it to happen like this. Things just started falling into place. I saw another way out of the situation with Estavez. A way for us to survive. Ethan, just listen—"

"Can you just—can you just give me a minute?" Ethan rose out of bed and walked to the giant sliding doors that framed out the private beach below him.

Jack stayed near the bed, silently watching him. The navy-colored waves were crashing silently against the shore below. It was still dark outside; he guessed it was maybe four or five in the morning.

Ethan tried to collect himself and calm his nerves. He

could feel his hands shaking. His whole body was reverberating with the news. The hangover from all the scotch he had consumed that evening was forming into a headache. The elegantly decorated room was hazy in the deep morning light. He needed a moment to clear the cobwebs from his brain and figure out how this was really happening. But he knew. Deep down, he felt certain if he turned to look behind him, he would see his brother. His brother who, maybe fifteen minutes ago, he'd thought he'd lost forever.

After a few minutes, Ethan turned to face him. "Okay, Jack. Tell me." The rattling sound of his own voice betrayed him. His emotions were of an elixir of rage and relief, swirling through his veins. His brother, whom he had loved and stood by his whole life, had betrayed him, lied to him, and hurt him in a way that he didn't even know how to begin to process.

Part of him wanted to run up and hug his brother, whom he'd barely been apart from his whole life. But when he thought Jack was dead, there was a little part of their relationship that had died too. It wasn't until he saw Jack alive that he realized it.

"Ethan, thank you. I mean, I'm sorry. I'm so sorry."

Jack walked toward him, reached out and grabbed Ethan, pulled him in for a hug. Ethan stiffly hugged him back. When he stepped away, he gave Ethan a unsure look. "Let's sit down," he said, gesturing to the round marble table flanked by four silver chairs.

Jack told Ethan the same story he had told Sydney about the crash and his rescue. "When I realized no one knew who I was, I saw an opportunity. I thought I could work behind the scenes and get us out of the deal with Estavez. The fisherman brought me to a port in Honduras. I had enough money on me to survive and scraped together a little bit more to get a laptop. That was all I needed to hack into the RicoCasino.com servers. I created a piece of code to skim small amounts of money—pennies on the dollar—into an offshore account. I still knew all the access codes, and because everyone thought I was dead, no one was looking for me." He took a deep breath and rubbed his hands on the cool marble. He looked up at Ethan. "It took me some time, but I was able to get enough money to pay off Estavez and even a little more. Just over two million dollars."

Ethan almost laughed. He couldn't believe it. Jack was smart and extremely talented with computers, but this was beyond what he thought Jack was capable of.

"So, you're telling me you stole money from Estavez— over two million dollars—and you want me to use that money to pay him back? With his own money?" Ethan finally let out a small laugh. "I thought he wanted me dead. Now he's gonna kill us both."

"I'm already dead," Jack said with a mischievous smile. Ethan was sure his face gave away his anger. The smile quickly disappeared. "What, too soon?"

He wanted to slug Jack again, but it was hard to stay mad at his brother. He settled for a dirty look. "Yeah, man, a little too soon," he said as he drummed his fingers on the table-top. "So, how do I get access to the money?"

"I've got everything set up and ready to go. I just need the account numbers to wire the money to." He paused for a moment, scratching the whiskers of his freshly grown beard.

"Listen, Ethan, there's something else."

"What?"

"I followed you yesterday, into Shettle Wood. I saw who you met with." Jack arched one eyebrow as he spoke. Ethan felt his throat tighten. "And we had a little conversation after you left." He reached down and pulled a small bottle out of his pocket. Ethan instantly recognized it as the same bottle he had purchased. He sat it on the table between them. "What were you planning to do with Rohypnol? Is this about Marissa's money?"

Ethan leaned back in his chair and took a deep breath. Had Jack asked him the same question six months ago, before his death, he would have told him everything. But now? He couldn't be trusted. Everything had changed between them. Ethan reached over and snatched the bottle off the table.

"It's none of your business," he said, pocketing the bottle into his lounge pants. Silence fell between the brothers, and they sat staring at each other in the hazy light. Ethan could hear the quiet rise and fall of the tide behind the sliding glass doors.

"Ethan," he began, a pleading look in his eyes, "this isn't like it was with Mom and Dad. We have other...options."

Ethan felt an anger spark in his chest. "How dare you bring them into this."

"Ethan, you know what I mean. It—"

"It was *your* idea. The fire was your idea, Jack. You just didn't have the guts to light the match."

Jack opened his mouth to speak and then shut it again. He looked out toward the ocean and then back at Ethan.

"It doesn't matter now," he said, shrugging his shoulders. "I've got the money. I just need the account numbers and—"

"Jack," he said, holding up his hand to silence him. "I appreciate everything you've done. Really, I can't believe you pulled this off without me. But paying off Estavez isn't going to stop him. He's only going to ask for more."

"Then I will find a way to get us more money."

"No," Ethan said, shaking his head. "It won't work. I have to marry Marissa tomorrow. Today. Estavez is here. And if I don't walk down that aisle, I'll be dead before I leave the island."

"He's here?" Jack said, a look of panic in his eyes.

"Yes."

Jack ran his hands through his hair, a gesture he always did when he was frustrated. Ethan sighed. There were so many gestures of Jack's that he knew so well. *Damnit, Jack.*

"The truth is you're too late," Ethan said. "I've already struck a deal with the FBI. I'm going to be wired up this morning, before the wedding. They want me to get Estavez to confess to Lizzy's murder. It's a done deal."

He stood up to signal that this was the end of the conversation. The look on Jack's face spoke volumes. He opened his mouth to speak and then shut it again. Finally he stood up. The brothers faced each other, bracing for the next move.

"Ethan...I just spent the last six months getting the money together to save your ass. You got us into this mess, remember? If you hadn't gambled away our profits, I wouldn't have had to scramble the money together in the first place." Ethan could see the color spreading across Jack's cheeks, an emotional cue he knew well. "And you're just going to ditch my plan and go with the feds? Just like that, end of discussion? If you think they'll let you work in online gambling ever again after this, you're fooling yourself."

"Did you discuss your plans with me when you decided to play dead? To leave me behind while you went off with some harebrained idea to get the money? I thought you were fucking dead, Jack!" He slammed his fist down on the table, nearly toppling it over. "But no, you had to go off and prove yourself just like you always wanted. Prove that you could make it without me. And look, you did it." He brushed an invisible speck of dirt off Jack's shoulder.

"I never wanted to do it without you, but it was the only way. It never would have worked if you had known I was alive. We would have been caught!" Jack was yelling now, his voice growing louder with each word he spat in Ethan's face.

"It doesn't matter! At least we would have been together." Ethan finally broke free from the face-off and strode to the door leading to the hallway. "I want you to leave. Go run back to Sydney, or fly off to your new home in South America, I don't care. But I don't want to be a part of your plan. And *I don't need your money.*" He emphasized the last five words, letting them hang in the still air.

Ethan stood at the door, his hand shaking as he reached for the handle. Jack stared at him, the shock registering on his face. Then his expression changed, and he furrowed his eyebrows. He took a few steps toward him and then suddenly broken into a run. As he lunged at Ethan, he angled his body downward, like a linebacker ready to deliver a heavy blow. He pummeled into Ethan with his shoulder and knocked him into the wall.

"I did it for you!" he screamed as they wrestled to the ground. The tension between them had finally reached a boiling point, and they spilled onto the floor. Jack landed himself on top of Ethan and pinned his arms to the ground with his legs. His first punch connected with Ethan's right jaw and Ethan felt the impact smash through the rest of his skull. Jack had always had a strong right hook, and Ethan knew he could only withstand a few punches from his brother before he blacked out.

He instinctively swung his legs to the side, trying to knock Jack off balance. It worked and as Jack fell back, Ethan freed himself and shoved him under the built-in bar. They were equally matched in height, although Ethan had more muscle and weight to work to his advantage. He used that to push his brother underneath the thick granite countertop, pinning him between the wall and a small drink refrigerator tucked beneath.

"You did it for yourself," Ethan said as he gripped Jack's neck, choking the air from his lungs. Jack was pushing against Ethan's forearm, trying to break his grip. Jack was only a few moments away from passing out. Ethan tried to stop himself from inflicting too much pain, but he felt a rage mixed with grief channeling itself from the center of his body down into his hands. Squeezing the life out of Jack was nearly cathartic. He knew he needed to stop before he did something he regretted, but he couldn't.

As he debated letting Jack go, he caught a flash of glass from one of the whiskey bottles scattered on the floor nearby. Jack seemed to notice it at the same time, proving their thinking was always in alignment even when they were at odds with each other. But in this case, Jack's body was positioned closest to the bottle. He let go of Ethan's forearm, just long enough to grab the neck of the long glass bottle and launch it toward Ethan's head.

The impact sent a searing blast of pain through his skull, straight from his right temple and sinking quickly to the back of his neck. His head was jolted to the side, and he could taste the tangy metal blood in his mouth. He fought to stay conscious as his body crumpled toward the ground.

As he began to pass out, his eyes fell on the garment bag hanging in his closet.

He could almost see the crisply pressed white tuxedo inside, the suit he was supposed to wear to his wedding.

THIRTY-THREE

SYDNEY

HOUSEKEEPING.

She could hear the word but it sounded far away as if she were at the bottom of a deep well and someone was speaking to her from the top. She started to stir, but when she did so, there was a tightening around her wrists and ankles. Her body tensed up. A gentle knock seemed to bring her into the room. She opened one eye and then her other. She realized she was on the floor.

"Oh, no!" she heard a women's voice shriek. "Ma'am, are you okay?"

As Sydney's eyes began to focus, she could see a black woman in a maid's uniform crouching over her. Sydney started to panic, when she realized there was a rope binding her arms and legs to the heavy wooden posts of the hotel bed.

"Um, I think so," she said. "Can you untie me?"

"Of course, of course," she replied. The woman began working frantically on the ropes. They had been tied tightly. She could see from the callouses on the woman's hands that she was used to hard work. The woman seemed to follow her eyes. "You are lucky," she said, giving her a reassuring smile. "My father was a fisherman. I am no stranger to untying knots."

After several minutes, Sydney was freed, and she pulled herself up into a sitting position. "Thank you," she said, squeezing the woman's shoulders.

"Do you want me to call someone, ma'am?"

Call someone? Sydney eyes widened as the memories rushed back to her. *Jack!*

That son of a bitch tied her up and left her in this room. Wherever this room was. She could tell by the décor that they were still on El Brillo Azul's property. *Thank goodness*, she thought. She looked around the room and saw a clock on the nightstand. It was 12:30 p.m.

The wedding!

The ceremony was to begin in thirty minutes, and she was still wearing her robe. She looked back at the maid.

"Oh no, no, I'm fine," she said, trying to give her a convincing smile. "My boyfriend and I just got a little carried away last night."

The woman made a face but then quickly smiled back. "Oh, okay."

"But thank you again," she said and touched her arm. This woman had no idea how truly grateful she was. "I've got to go, now. Goodbye."

Sydney jumped to her feet and raced out the door. As she padded barefoot down the hallway, she tried to get her bearings. She had a minor headache, but other than that, she seemed to be fine. Jack hadn't hurt her. *Physically, anyway*, she thought.

As she reached the end of the hallway, she found a property map and located the honeymoon section. From there she practically ran back to her room.

As she opened the door, she was relieved to see it was empty. She definitely had no time to explain to Alex where she had been. That was a story for later. She quickly went to the closet and pulled out the pale blue bridesmaid's dress Marissa had Vera Wang design for the wedding. As she slipped the one-shouldered gown over her head, she heard a banging on the door.

"Sydney, are you in there?" She heard the familiar voice of Jessica, the wedding planner, on the other side.

"Yes! Be right there!" she said as she zipped the gown up the bottom half of her back. She pulled open the door and found herself face-to-face with a very unhappy-looking woman.

"Sydney! We've been looking everywhere for you!"

"I know, it's a long story. I—"

Jessica cut her off with a wave of her hand. "Let's save story time for later. I need you to finish your makeup and be out in the hallway in five minutes! I'll be waiting!"

"Got it," Sydney said and let the door shut as she dashed into the bathroom. It was truly time to put her five-minute makeup routine to the test. She was moving so quickly she barely had time to process what Jack had done.

As she dashed out into the hallway, she found Jessica waiting for her, a clipboard in one arm. When she saw Sydney emerge from the room, she tapped the earpiece of the black headset she was wearing.

"Okay, I've got her. We're on our way," she heard her say. Jessica didn't say a word to Sydney, just gave her a sharp nod, indicating she was to follow her. She stayed a few steps ahead of her, chattering nonstop on her headset as they walked quickly toward the ceremony.

As the sounds of their footsteps clattered down the hallway, Sydney thought of her own wedding. When she and

Jack had married on a beach with just a few people, barefoot in the sand, she had barely worn any makeup, and they were both casually dressed as if their next stop was a summer barbeque.

It was a distinct contrast to the scene that unfolded in front of her as they rounded the corner. The wedding setup was nothing short of glamorous. Crisp white chairs were lined up in perfectly straight rows, punctuated with several gorgeous bouquets of white lilies, magnolias, carnations, and flowers Sydney didn't even know the names of. A long white silk runner snaked down the center aisle and landed under a massive structure built of rustic beach limbs, more white flowers, and elegant greens that were suspended in the air between small twinkling crystals. It was a breathtaking sight, something you'd find flipping through a bridal magazine. Beyond the beautiful setup, the ocean waves rolled forward and back beneath a blue sky without a cloud in sight. If there had been a storm last night, Sydney had slept through it.

There were probably two hundred guests seated, which Marissa likely had to cut down to just close friends since she ran in large social circles. Sydney was sure that the people who did make the cut were honored to be there.

A small girl with bright blond curls bounced along the silken pathway dropping white rose petals along the way. Sydney watched her and silently wished she had a little girl of her own. She certainly had planned to have kids someday. It was odd that the thought occurred to her now, when her life seemed to be in the midst of chaos. But it was another one of the dreams she had to let go of when she lost Jack. Or at least, thought she lost him. *Damn it, Jack.*

She tried to refocus on the present. *Get through the wedding and life goes back to normal. Whatever the hell normal is at this point.* If she could stay the course and see the wedding through, she could take her time figuring out her next steps on the other end. And hopefully Jack would be out of her life for good.

After a long line of bridesmaids and groomsmen had made their way to the altar, it was Sydney's turn. She took the arm of Marissa's cousin, whose name she couldn't remember, and made her way toward the altar. Ethan was standing dutifully at the end of the path. She wondered what the conversation between him and Alex had been like the night before. She also wondered if Jack had revealed to his brother yet that he was alive and well. The thought of Jack made her feel queasy. She aimed her body straight ahead and told herself to keep putting one foot in front of the other.

As she walked closer to the altar, she made eye contact with Ethan. Something was off; she felt it right away. He seemed to be uncomfortable, shifting his weight from side to side and cracking his neck. Then he had his arms crossed in front of him, sliding one hand over the other nervously. His suit, a crisp white tuxedo, looked as if it were made for someone about twenty pounds heavier. She was surprised Marissa and Jessica would have allowed him to get away with such an untailored-looking fit.

She looked away from Ethan for a moment and scanned the crowd for Alex. She desperately hoped he was here. She needed his support. She felt safer when he was around.

And maybe she just liked having him there, because she liked *him.* You're not supposed to fall for the FBI agent who is helping clear you of any fraudulent involvement in an international crime ring. She realized then that if she didn't tell Alex about her meeting with Jack the night before, it might make her look suspicious, very suspicious actually.

She vowed to tell him everything as soon as the wedding was over.

There was no sign of Alex in the crowd, but as she peered into the groom's side of the aisle, her eyes caught on a white fedora with a sleek black band. The man looked distinctly Latin, with dark hair and hazel eyes she could barely make out in the sunlight. A gorgeous woman with long black hair sat next to him. He seemed to be studying the groom, intently.

That has to be Vincente Estavez. The thought made her blood run cold.

She shifted her gaze back to the altar and noticed that Ethan had several cuts on his neck, as if he had shaved too quickly and nicked himself. Trying not to be obvious, she glanced over her shoulder at him as she walked to her appointed place on the right side of the altar.

And then she knew, instantly. It wasn't Ethan standing there under the massive canopy of flowers awaiting his bride.

It was Jack.

THIRTY-FOUR

ETHAN

THE FIRST THING Ethan saw when he woke that morning was the large rain showerhead looming over him. He tried to move, but every muscle in his body was screaming at him to stay still. Not to mention, his head was throbbing.

Why was he on the shower floor? The way the light was shining through a tiny crack in the room let him know it was no longer early morning.

The wedding! The thought smacked him in the face and despite his pain he told his body to move.

At that point, he realized that he was tied up. *Jack, you son of bitch.* Jack had used a thick yellow rope to tie his hands and feet together. Hog-tied is what they called it as kids. When they were boys, they used to think it was funny to tie each other up and see who could escape. The problem was that Jack was always better at securing him in the ropes.

A sequence of thoughts flashed through his mind. *Where the heck did Jack get the rope? Did he bring it with him? Did he always know that he would tie up Ethan and try to stop the wedding?*

He brushed those thoughts aside. Right now, it didn't

matter why. He would ask Jack later, right before he punched that winning smile right off his face. What mattered now was getting out of this room as quickly as possible.

His body ached and he could see bruises on his arms and legs. He could only imagine what his face looked like. He could feel a pulsing pain at his right temple and in his swollen cheek. Luckily he could see just fine, well enough to spot his carry-on bag in the corner of the room. It took several minutes, but he was able to caterpillar himself toward the bag. He moved his hands up close enough to the front pouch, which held his car keys. The keys to his Range Rover were just a fob, but he had a condo key that was the perfect tool to loosen the ropes around his ankle.

Fifteen minutes later, Ethan was free of his bonds. He took a quick assessment of his face in the mirror. Not a pretty sight. He had a long gash on the side of his head. Nothing deep, but it was swollen and matted with blood. He grabbed a towel, washed the wound, and did the best he could with the tools he had. When he looked in the mirror again, he was satisfied. *Good enough to get married*, he thought. But certainly not good enough for the wedding photos. They could work that out later.

He dashed out into his suite, still a complete wreck from the night before. Two chairs near the balcony were flipped over next to a table that was on its side. There were liquor bottles scattered across the floor, and Ethan wondered for a second which bottle had put the gash in his head.

He reach the closet and pulled out the black garment bag that held his tuxedo. He'd had a special fitting before they left for the trip and the suit fit him like a glove. He pulled it off the hanging rack and tossed it on the bed nearby.

Ethan stopped. When he looked down at the bag, the zipper was hanging wide open. A gaping hole that revealed a deep fear in his chest. His suit was gone. Which from a lifetime of living with his brother meant one thing.

Damnit, Jack!

Marissa was probably saying her vows right now *to the wrong person*. He knew that once he told Jack that Estavez would kill him if he didn't marry Marissa, Jack would do everything in his power to protect him. Even if that meant standing in his place at the ceremony. Jack always had his back, even when they were fighting.

You've gone too far this time, brother.

Ethan found an extra set of clothes, dressed himself, and rushed to the door. But before he headed out into the sunlight, he turned back and grabbed something from underneath his mattress.

A gun.

THIRTY-FIVE

SYDNEY

THE VOICES inside Sydney's head were screaming so loudly, she was sure someone would hear them. She stole a few more looks at the man standing just ten feet from her, and sure enough it was Jack. Yes, Jack and Ethan were identical twins, but there were some subtle differences between them. Differences that only someone who spent a significant amount of time with them would notice. The way they stood, the nervous way that Jack tucked his hair behind his ears. The subtle difference in their hairlines, their posture.

Had they been standing side by side, you could see the differences. But in this case, everyone present assumed Jack was dead, so they had no reason to believe that the person at the altar was anyone other than Ethan.

This can't be happening.

Sydney's mind raced as quickly as her heart was beating. While the tropical breezes coming from the crashing waves behind them kept everyone else cool, Sydney's pale blue chiffon dress was becoming heavy and damp beneath her long wavy hair.

She looked out into the crowd. No one looked a bit

suspicious. The rows of chairs held only a sea of smiling faces. *If only they knew!*

Sydney stared down at the elegant bouquet of flowers she was clutching with white-knuckled fists. *I've got to stop this. I won't let Jack do this to Marissa.*

But what could she do? If she called out Jack right there in front of everyone, it would be a huge embarrassment for Marissa. Should she wait and signal her once she made it down the aisle? Would Marissa notice something was off, that Ethan didn't look like himself? No, Sydney had to stop things now. She began to step toward Jack.

But before she could move another foot forward in the sand, the pianist behind her began to play Pachelbel's "Canon in D Major." Everyone in the audience stood and turned. Sydney followed their stares and saw Marissa coming straight down the aisle.

Sydney felt like she had swallowed one of the large seashells that were displayed all around her. She held her breath to try and stop the tears from exploding down her cheeks. How could Jack do this? She finally looked at him. He was staring at Marissa, sweating profusely and clearly uncomfortable.

When Marissa finally made it to the altar, Jack reached forward and took her hands. Marissa let go and tried to push her veil toward him. Jack looked confused. Sydney wished she could see Marissa's face, but her position behind her only gave her a view of Jack.

"Veil," she heard Marissa whisper loudly. Jack finally took the hint and raised the veil up over her face. The netting caught on one of her earrings, and he fumbled with it, causing the crowd to stir with awkward laughter. Jack looked at the people and smiled. That's when she heard Marissa whisper under her breath. It was so soft—

unless you were a few feet next to her, you wouldn't have caught it.

"Jack?"

She knows.

The wedding officiant began to babble away, welcoming the people gathered in front of them. Sydney could not take her eyes off Jack's face. He was trying to force a smile on his lips and kept furrowing his eyebrows at Marissa as if she was saying something to him. He was softly shaking his head from side to side, trying to tell her to keep quiet.

The appointed minister began to speak the familiar words. "Do you, Marissa, take this man—"

Marissa turned her head to the minister and stopped him. "I'm sorry, I can't." She turned her head back to Jack and said, "How could you do this to me?"

She threw the large bouquet she was carrying on the ground and turned around to face Sydney.

"I'm sorry, I didn't know he would..." Sydney began, breathlessly.

Marissa met her gaze with a shocked stare and then narrowed her eyes again.

"Did you know? Did you know Jack was alive?"

"Just last night. Marissa, I'm sorry..."

Marissa didn't wait to hear what she had to say. She picked up the hem of her long white dress and started walking quickly down the center aisle. It was an odd sight to see all the heads in the room turn again in perfect unison and watch her as she stumbled forward. Jack looked over at Sydney.

"What the hell were you thinking?" she said, glaring at him.

Jack seemed to be frozen in place as if he wasn't sure what his next move should be. He finally turned his face from hers and started looking over the crowd, landing directly where Estavez had been sitting. Sydney followed his gaze. While everyone else was watching Marissa charge down the aisle, the two seats where Estavez and the beautiful Latin woman had been remained empty.

Estavez was gone.

Jack looked back at Sydney. He then stepped forward and leaned closely to whisper in her ear.

"Sydney, I'm sorry about last night. I didn't want you to get hurt. There is so much more I have to tell you." His eyes seemed to convey that he was speaking the truth, but Sydney knew she couldn't trust him. "But right now, I need to get out of here."

Jack started walking down the aisle, following the same path Marissa had just stumbled down moments ago. When he arrived at the end of the row of carefully decorated chairs, he took a sharp left turn and began to run.

Sydney watched him go, too stunned by the entire scene to move. When he was out of sight, the crowd began to whisper and murmur. She could see everyone looking around, watching for what might happen next. She saw several people had taken out their cell phones to film the entire incident.

Sydney finally threw down her bouquet and started after Jack. It was most likely the worst idea to follow him, but if she didn't get down to the truth of what had happened, she couldn't live with herself.

Messy, imperfect or not, she was finally ready to hear the truth.

THIRTY-SIX
SYDNEY

SYDNEY REACHED the edge of the beach and stopped to locate Jack. She couldn't see him, her eyes being blinded by the bright sun and maybe even the blood that was pumping through her veins at breakneck speed.

Where is he going? she wondered. She looked from left to right, sweeping across the broad white concrete structures dotted with perfectly coifed bushes and palm trees reaching skyward. The hotel complex was fairly quiet once you had some distance between the wedding guests and the rest of the hotel. It seemed everyone who was either staying or working at the hotel was attending the lavish wedding.

She looked across the wide beach and saw several crushed gravel pathways snaking between the buildings. She wondered if he was going back to find Ethan. It was then that a thought popped into her head: *where is Ethan?*

Surely Ethan did not give Jack his permission to impersonate him on his wedding day. Or was this a step in their dim-witted plan? Either way, Sydney knew that Ethan was staying in a bachelor suite at the north side of the complex and headed in that direction.

Her instincts had served her well because as soon as she rounded the next building she saw Jack walking briskly down one of the gravel paths.

"Jack! Wait!" she cried between breaths. Whether or not he heard her, he kept moving forward, into a deep tangle of trees, shrubs, and grasses that looked like a small jungle. It seemed her daily regime of workout classes was working in her favor, because she was quickly closing the distance between them.

Had Sydney been focused on anything else but Jack, she would have noticed that there was also someone closing some distance on her. As she geared up to call after Jack again, she felt a firm hand around her upper bicep.

"Sydney! Hold on." She whirled around to see Alex standing slightly breathless behind her. She noticed he was sweating and in his other hand was a gun.

"Alex, let me go! I'm going to lose him."

"It's dangerous. We don't know where Ethan is going. Let me handle this."

"That's not Ethan!" she screamed. Alex stood back, giving her a look you'd give a crazy person.

"What do you mean?"

"It's Jack! Jack is alive. He found me last night after the rehearsal dinner. I was going to tell you, I just—"

"So you spent the night with him?"

"No, no that's not what happened. He drugged me and tied me up in his room." Alex made a face as if he was not convinced. "Trust me, I'm telling the truth."

Alex sighed. "I've been looking everywhere for you. I was worried they'd gotten to you."

"I'm fine." She was touched by his concern, but the sentiment would have to wait. "But we need to catch Jack. He's getting away."

"Wait, so that was Jack at the altar, not Ethan?"

"Yes," she said, trying to pull him in the direction Jack had been walking. She could almost see the news settle into his mind as he processed what she was saying.

"Why?"

"I don't know, but I'm going to find out the truth. Please, let's go."

"Okay, but stay close to me." Alex pulled a gun from underneath his jacket. He was wearing a khaki linen suit with a skinny tie, apparently dressed for the wedding. Sydney wondered why she hadn't seen him there. He grabbed Sydney's hand, and they began to run into the thick foliage, following the path Jack had been walking on just moments earlier.

As the path led deeper into the junglelike brush and farther away from the resort, Sydney began to get even more nervous. Alex had pulled his weapon, and the emotions of the situation were running high. What would Alex do to Jack once they reached him?

She was about to find out because when they rounded the next corner there was a sudden break in the trees and Jack was walking just about twenty feet in front of them.

"Jack!" Sydney yelled out to him. He kept walking.

"FBI," cried Alex. "Don't move."

Jack came to a dead stop.

THIRTY-SEVEN

ETHAN

WITH HIS HEART RACING, Ethan ran down the hallway of the resort. He could hear the sound of his own breathing and his heavy footsteps as he clattered down the hallway but little else. The hotel was unusually quiet, devoid of the busy guests typically milling around hallways.

As he made his way clear of the white stucco buildings, he could see the wedding setup spread out over the edge of the beach. Hundreds of white chairs in long rows with chattering guests. He squinted in the bright sun, trying to see if he could make out Jack at the altar. A pair of sunglasses would have come in handy. Then he realized that many of the guests were looking at each other instead of facing the altar and talking in hushed tones. Something must have happened to Jack. *Of course*, he thought, *surely Marissa would know it wasn't me.*

He took two more steps in the direction of the wedding circus and then stopped. He saw Sydney running north toward the pathway that led into the lush jungle surrounding the complex. He could see Alex running after her, just a few steps away from reaching her.

Ethan had a fairly good idea of where they were going. The dense jungle had a path that led north, away from the resort, to another private beach area. If Jack needed to make a quiet exit from the hotel without being seen, that was the way to go.

Ethan quickly stepped behind a massive palm tree that had been wrapped in twinkling lights. He didn't want to be seen. Placing his hand on his gun, as if to reassure himself, he waited at least thirty seconds before tailing them.

He tried to stay calm as the adrenaline ripped through his body. He stepped onto the gravel pathway and tried to focus on what his options were. He was furious with Jack. How could he do this to him, his own brother? It was actually difficult to think, as his head was still throbbing from the glass bottle that Jack had struck him in the head with. The intense heat and humidity from the trees caused him to start sweating profusely, which didn't help either.

Jack had managed to screw up every part of Ethan's plan. Once Estavez found out Jack was alive, he wouldn't hesitate to kill them both, the first chance he got. And to make matters worse, Ethan had now blown any chance he had of working with the FBI. Even if he cut a deal with them to bring down Estavez, he knew there was no way they'd let him keep his business. He'd lost his best chance at leverage.

As he wiped the sweat from his eyes and picked up his pace, one thing become clear: he was going to kill Jack, if Estavez didn't get to him first.

THIRTY-EIGHT

SYDNEY

THERE WAS an eerie silence among the three of them, as Sydney watched Jack standing with his back to her and Alex. The space where they had caught up with Jack was densely lined with palm trees and tropical green shrubs that reached out over the pathway as if trying to grab hold of the passersby. The sun was filtering through the palm branches above them, which gave them some respite from the Caribbean heat. She glanced sideways at Alex, wondering what his next move was.

Alex had his gun drawn and was pointing it at Jack. He was laser-focused, breathing slowly. "Please turn around."

Hands still held in the air, Jack slowly turned his body toward the two of them. When he had managed to position himself facing them, Sydney caught sight of his expression. She obviously didn't know Jack like she thought she did, but she knew enough to recognize his emotional state. Anger, bordering on rage.

He had managed to undo the his bow tie. It now dangled from his neck, which was red and wet from the heat. He managed to change his expression and gave Alex a half smile. He refused to look at Sydney. "Have I done something wrong?"

Alex kept his gaze steady, unflinching. "That depends. Can you tell me what your name is?"

He didn't hesitate. "Jack Evans."

Alex took a deep breath and slightly shifted his weight from one leg to another but kept his arm extended toward Jack. "Mr. Evans, my name is Alex Birch. I am an agent with the FBI. Are you aware you've broken a host of laws by faking your own death?"

"If I remember correctly, it's not illegal to fake your own death. And anyway, I wasn't faking my death. I was lost and no one has been looking for me. I couldn't find my way back to the U.S."

"You're lying, Jack," said Sydney. She couldn't bear to stay silent another moment. She took several steps toward him, nearly stumbling over her gown—somewhere in the path behind her she had kicked off her nude pumps, leaving the hemline too long in the front. "When will you stop lying? You can't run away and hide like you did before. You need to face your problems."

"Face my problems?" he said, finally turning his eyes toward her. "I wasn't running, Sydney. I had a plan to get us all out of this mess. You, me, Ethan, Marissa. No one seems to understand what I was trying to accomplish." He looked again at Alex. "May I put my hands down now?"

"No. You'll put your hands down when I say it's okay to do so," Alex replied, rearranging the grip on his gun.

"I'm still not quite clear on why you have a gun on me. I haven't been charged with anything, nor have I done anything wrong. You need to let me go."

"I can't do that," said Alex.

"Listen, man, I'm going to put my hands down slowly. No

funny business, okay?" Jack began to slowly lower his hands. Sydney was looking between Jack and Alex, holding her breath. Alex was stone-faced, not making another move. Once his hands had reached his side, he let out a slow breath.

"Okay, listen, man. This is going to get really ugly in a minute if Estavez finds us." He looked over Alex's shoulder. "I can see that you don't have any backup nearby. And I guarantee Estavez isn't coming alone." He paused as if to make his point. "You need to let me go."

Sydney could see the recognition of the words fall over Alex's face. He shifted his weight again, the sound of his shoes crunching over the gravel.

At that moment, a buzzing noise began to ring out from Jack's pocket. He looked down. "I need to take this," he said.

"Not a chance, buddy," Alex said, laying another cold stare in his direction.

"Jack, don't do it," said Sydney.

He looked directly at her.

"Sydney, you need to get out of here. Things are going to get ugly. Estavez is going to come looking for me as soon as he realizes what happened. If I don't leave now, I'm as good as dead. And so are you."

"I'm not leaving until you tell me why the hell you did all this. Why did you pretend to be Ethan on his wedding day?"

"We got into a fight last night," he said, wiping the sweat from his forehead. Alex tensed and repositioned his gun. "He didn't take the news that I was alive very well. Things got heated and Ethan got hurt. He wasn't able to make it to the wedding, so I took his place."

"But why? And did you really think that Marissa wouldn't know it was you?"

Jack shrugged. She could see rings of sweat forming underneath his arms.

"It wasn't a perfect plan, but what choice did I have? If Ethan didn't marry Marissa, Estavez would have killed him before he left the island."

"Where is Ethan now?" Alex said, keeping his gun steady on Jack as he spoke.

Jack seemed to be looking beyond Alex and into the jungle. "Where he always is: trailing behind me."

After that, it all seemed to happen in slow motion. A loud bang came from the bushes about twenty feet behind her. There was a loud thump in the underbrush and the sound of someone skidding onto the gravel pathway. Alex grabbed Sydney's right arm to pull her down to the ground, but they tumbled helplessly over each other and landed in the dirt. As she caught a glimpse of Jack falling backward , she noticed a bright right blotch of blood soaking his crisp white tuxedo.

THIRTY-NINE

ETHAN

"JACK!" Sydney cried out as he fell to the ground.

Ethan could see a soda can–sized blood spot on Jack's white tuxedo, just below his right shoulder blade. He was aiming to injure but not kill him. Jack was lying unconscious on the ground; the heat mixed with the shock of the blast must have knocked him out for a moment.

Ethan immediately went after Alex's gun, which had fallen to the ground when he grabbed Sydney. Alex tried to reach forward and capture it before Ethan reached it, but it was too late. Ethan shoved the gun into his trousers.

He held the gun extended at Alex's head and took a step back.

"Get up," he said.

"Ethan, don't do this," Alex said as he slowly regained his footing. "We had a deal."

"And I was prepared to honor that deal," Ethan replied, not taking his gun off the agent. "But there's been a change of plans. My brother has managed to mess things up, again."

Ethan could see a small bulge in Alex's right pant leg. Probably another gun. "I need you to keep your hands in the air, please," he said, drawing his eyes from Alex's face to his pant pocket. "No funny business."

Alex nodded in agreement. He took several steps back, away from Ethan, and looked down at Sydney.

At the same time, Jack began to stir. He sat up and grabbed his shoulder, grunting in pain. He looked up at Ethan, glaring.

"You shot me," he said, a look of hurt and shock registering on his face.

"I couldn't let you leave me again," Ethan said, all the adrenaline coursing through his veins leaving his words thick in his mouth. "Leave me in another mess. Estavez is going to kill me for what you did. And I'm not going to ace him alone."

He saw Jack start to get up and reach for something behind his back. Thinking quickly, Ethan reached down and grabbed Sydney, who had been sitting motionless on the ground to his left, probably trying to figure out what to do. In one swift movement, he wrapped his arm around her neck and pushed the gun to her head.

"Don't even think about it."

FORTY

SYDNEY

SYDNEY FELT the gun pressing hard against her temple. She could feel Ethan shaking slightly as he faced off with Jack.

How the hell did I get in the middle of this? she wondered.

She would have said something, but Ethan held her so tightly, she could barely breathe let alone speak.

Jack was staring at the both of them, his eyes wide with fear. That expression, that look of panic in his eyes, made her question everything she believed up to that point. Maybe he had really done this for her? She could see the beads of sweat on his face, neck, and even his hands. The once crisp white suit, now muddled with dark patches of moisture, clung to his skin. A lone lock of hair was sticking to his forehead and hanging over his left eye. He didn't dare move a muscle to swipe it free.

Alex was now standing just a few feet from Jack, facing Sydney and Ethan. It would seem to anyone watching that Alex and Jack had gone from opposing teams to rooting for the same cause: her safety.

Her relationship with Ethan had always been a little

tense. She felt Ethan's resentment when she swooped in and garnered all of Jack's attention. The twins had always been close, even after she and Jack had married, but it wasn't the same. The space between them seemed to widen, allowing Sydney to fulfill many of the roles that Ethan was used to playing: confidant, cheerleader, partner, source of joy.

But even though she and Ethan had never been close, threatening her life seemed to take things to a level beyond what she could have imagined. The different ways this situation could go fanned out in front of her, and salty tears mixed with her own sweat trailed down her cheeks. Based on all of the Netflix series she'd binge-watched since Jack's death, the next thing that needed to happen was for her to elbow Ethan in the stomach and break free, letting someone else have a chance to pull a gun on Ethan. Unfortunately for her, things didn't quite happen that way.

Jack broke the tension. "Ethan, what are you doing? You're not going to shoot Sydney."

Ethan didn't move, his feet planted firmly in the gravel below. "Try me."

A look of surprise mixed with fear broke across Jack's face. "Okay, fine. What do you want?"

"I want you to face Estavez with me. I'm not taking the fall alone."

Jack sighed deeply. He looked down at the ground and then up again at Ethan. He lowered his hand briefly to swipe the wet lock of hair out of his eyes. "Ethan, you know I can't do that. He will kill me. I've got the money you owe him. Just let me wire the funds, and then you can work out a deal—"

"I already struck a deal, a deal that was going to cost me...a lot. Everything I had left. But it gave me a chance to start over. If I use your money, stolen money, I'll be looking over my back for the rest of my life. I'll never be able to rest."

Jack took a step closer to them, leaving Alex behind him. His demeanor seemed to change, as if he was about ready to deal a blow.

"So what exactly was your plan, Ethan? Before Alex here showed up and offered you a deal with the feds, how were you going to pay off Estavez without a dime to your name? And why did this plan coincide with the wedding?"

Sydney felt Ethan's entire body go rigid. He tightened his grip around her neck, causing her to gasp for air. *What was Jack getting at?* She knew that Marissa was in trouble, but she didn't think it had anything to do with Ethan. She thought it was more about Estavez hurting her.

"It doesn't matter now," Ethan said through clenched teeth, as if warning Jack to keep his mouth shut.

"I know the way you think, Ethan. You don't have to pretend with me. Does Marissa know about the fire? About our parents?"

"Shut up, Jack."

"Like you said, I wasn't the one who lit the match. Because despite everything they did to us, I still loved them. But with you it was different. You could turn your feelings off like a switch."

"I did it to protect you," Ethan said, loosening his grip just a bit. Sydney gulped in some fresh air.

"You did it for yourself. Just like when you gambled away all of our profits. Just like how you planned to roofie your own wife and dump her off the side of the yacht you rented for the honeymoon."

Ethan's grip tightened again around her throat.

"Yes, I figured it out. I'm your twin, remember? We're connected. I tried to do everything I could to save you," Jack said, holding a hand over his bleeding shoulder. "But you still managed to screw that up because you always want more. You can't see past your own greed."

With each word, Jack inched closer and closer to the spot where Ethan was holding her. She noticed he made a quick eye movement as if he saw something behind her.

"I had it handled, Jack, *without you.* Don't come any closer or your precious Sydney is going to have a hole in her pretty little head."

She felt the tension around her throat suddenly release, and she sucked up the air around her with a fierce breath. It happened so fast, Sydney didn't have any time to react. She stood there nearly motionless. As she reached for her throat to feel for damage, she heard a loud crack and saw Ethan crumpling in a pile next to her. She took two steps forward and made an about-face.

Standing in front of her now, just a few feet away, was Marissa. She was still wearing her wedding dress, which was damp and covered in brown patches from the dirt path. Her makeup was smeared, dark drips of mascara running down her face, giving her a gothic look. But what caught Sydney by surprise was the massive silver vase she held in her hands. She realized that Jack must have seen her coming and had kept Ethan talking while Marissa got close enough to deliver the blow.

"Sydney, are you okay?" Marissa said breathlessly.

"Marissa, you...you just saved my life," she said as she ran to her friend and embraced her. Marissa's small frame was shaking. "Thank you," she whispered in her ear.

Sydney then heard the sound of feet scrambling behind her. She turned again to see Jack running farther down the path and into the jungle, Alex lunging after him. She looked back at Marissa.

"Go!" Marissa cried. "I've got the FBI coming right behind me."

She was right. Sydney caught sight of some armed officers in black uniforms arrive on the scene with Marissa and Ethan as she again began to run down the path, following Jack and Alex.

FORTY-ONE

SYDNEY

SYDNEY COULD FEEL trickles of water running down her face as she bounded after the two men. One from her past, and possibly one whom she had a future with? That was yet to be determined, but she didn't want Jack to get hurt. Truthfully, she didn't know what she wanted, and as her heart pounded, she realized she was tired of chasing after him.

As she ran farther into the jungle, she realized she was falling too far behind them. The sounds of the two men running seemed to get farther and farther away, until all she could hear was the frogs and birds singing from the trees. She realized she would never catch them and stopped to take a breath.

Her throat was still burning from Ethan nearly strangling her. She placed her hands lightly on her knee caps and leaned over to take some deep, soothing breaths. Although the adrenaline was still pumping through her veins, she was growing tired.

After a few moments, she stood up straight. She looked at the path in front of her that seemed to be leading to the other side of the island, and then behind her, where she had left Marissa and Ethan alone on the pathway.

Her own path had narrowed considerably and was now just wide enough for one person to walk on. She had small red lashes on her upper arms from sharp palm fronds slapping against her as she ran.

Sydney had two choices at this point: she could run after Alex and Jack, or go back and help her friend. Marissa could clearly handle herself and she was impressed with her friend's reflexes. Just as she was about to make her decision, she heard a loud pop on the path in front of her. Without thinking she began to run again toward Alex and Jack.

Finally, she could see sunlight shining through the green-lined archway—the end of the path. She took another step and her foot caught on something large and warm on the ground below her. The ground rose up to meet her as she tumbled forward in a ball of blue silk and chiffon layers. Looking around to see what had caused her fall, she saw Alex laying on his side, with his hand clutching his ear. Blood was seeping through the gaps in his fingers.

"Alex! Oh my god, are you okay?"

Alex squinted in her direction and grunted in pain. "I'm fine, he just shot my ear."

"You are not fine!" Sydney said and she crawled toward him. "Here, let me help." A few years of Girl Scouts had prepared Sydney for a variety of situations. She reached under a few layers of her dress and ripped out enough silk to make a dressing for his wound. Alex watched her work, trying to pretend he was fine, but he was clearly in a lot of pain. Sydney managed to gather enough silk to wrap the dressing around his head several times before tying it in a knot. A red splat of blood quickly soaked through the side of her creation, but it was the best she could do for now.

"Come on," she said, pulling Alex's arm, "we need to find someone who can help us. And you need a hospital."

Alex looked at her as he steadied himself. He was having trouble getting his footing, and she wondered how much blood he had lost.

"He got away, Sydney. I couldn't stop him."

She looked ahead toward the beach as they pulled themselves free of the jungle's brush. The light hit them both, and they had to squint to see anything in the bright light. Sydney took a quick look around and saw no sign of Jack.

"Don't worry," she said, putting her arm around Alex's waist. "He'll be back. If not for me, he will definitely want to finish the fight with his brother."

FORTY-TWO

ETHAN

ETHAN TRIED to open his eyes, but the searing pain in his head made it hard to do so. He could hear the chattering of voices around him, mostly with Jamaican accents. He tenderly lifted his head. Small pieces of gravel were sticking to his left cheek and temple. But movement of any kind was too much of an effort. He felt his arms being roughly pulled behind his back, and he heard the click of stainless-steel handcuffs as they pushed against his wrists.

Truthfully any distraction from the pain in his head was welcome. He was drowsy and disoriented. He tried to recall what had happened since Jack had stood before him, chiding him about his plan to take Marissa's money. How had Jack figured out his plans? The pain in his head was too much to think about anything for more than a split second. The last memory he had was of a searing pain at the back of his skull and then he was falling.

He started to open his eyes as he was pulled up to a sitting position. He felt a punch of nausea hit his stomach, and he was able to lean forward just far enough to prevent vomiting all over himself. He felt someone nearby reach down and prop him up until he stopped. He was certain he had a concussion, having been knocked unconscious twice in one day. There was no way he could stand. He was sweating and freezing at the same time, and he felt his body shaking. His vision become blurry again, and he was able to make out a stained white gown and a stretcher heading in his direction before he passed out again.

He went in and out of sleep for the next few hours. When he finally became conscious again, a dimly lit hospital room came into view. By the lackluster paint peeling from the walls, he guessed he was still in Jamaica.

He started to get up and realized that he was wearing handcuffs that chained him to the hospital bed. He tugged and pulled for several seconds before realizing there was no use. Exhausted and still woozy from the multiple blows to his head, he fell back onto the pillows propped behind his head.

He looked to his right and realized a large man was seated next to him. He was hunched over, his massive shoulders nearly blocking out the light from the only window in the room. He watched Ethan with an intensity that made him squirm in his bed.

"Good morning, Mr. Evans," he said with a deep, guttural voice. "Glad to have you back with us. My name is Inspector Sam O'Connell. I'd like to ask you a few questions."

FORTY-THREE
SYDNEY

SYDNEY SHIFTED HER POSITION AGAIN, causing the vinyl seat cover of her chair to creak and moan in the corner. The light from the room gently filtered through the sheer curtains. She could hear voices coming and going down the hallway and the gentle *beep-beep* of the heart-rate monitor next to the bed.

She had been waiting three hours for Alex to wake up from his ear surgery. After they left the beach, they had quickly found a nearby resort and the staff called for an ambulance. It was the first time Sydney had ridden in an ambulance since she was a kid, and the experience in Jamaica was no different. Alex took the ride in stride, although she could see by the grimace on his face that he was in pain.

And now she was waiting. The first hour she had spent quietly looking out the window at the rolling hills and mist hanging on to the valleys below. She looked at it as a type of meditation, a chance to reflect on everything that happened. It wasn't long after though that her phone began to beep and vibrate, beckoning her from her quiet respite and back to the realities of the world.

Marissa had texted to let her know she was safe. She was preparing to fly out tomorrow and wanted Sydney to join her. She wouldn't take no for an answer. When Sydney was ready, all she had to do was call the number and a private car service would pick her up. She had never taken a private jet before and was actually looking forward to the experience.

Once she had pulled out her phone to text Marissa, she realized she had an inbox jammed with messages. Part of her wanted to delete every app and social media account on her phone, a sharp digression from the way she had felt before the last few days.

She posted a few outfit photos to her Instagram feed, responded to several emails from brands she worked with, posted an update on her Facebook page, but it all felt empty. She felt disconnected with the rest of the world, like the rose-colored glasses through which she saw her social media presence had been ripped away.

She heard Alex stirring from the other end of the room. He was lying in a white hospital bed, sheets tucked in tight so as not to disturb the web of cords and wires surrounding his bed. There was a thick white gauze bandage wrapped several times around his head with a bulge around his right ear. The color from days in the sun had drained from his face, and she worried he had lost some of his sparkle. She moved closer to him as his eyes fluttered open.

"Alex?" she whispered into his good ear.

He looked at her. A smile creased the corners of his mouth and when he saw her, she could have sworn she saw the color come back into his face. The sparkle was still there.

"Sydney, what are you doing here?"

"I just wanted to make sure you were okay. How are you feeling?"

His squinted a bit and tried to move. "I'm a bit stiff, but I'll live."

"Good," she said with a satisfied smile. "Good news or bad news first?"

"I could handle some good news right now." She paused, leaned in, and placed her hand on his.

"Well, the good news is, I spoke with the doctor and they were able to save your ear. With some therapy, your hearing should come back as well. Full recovery."

"Bad?" he said, grabbing her hand in his.

"Your boss is here, Inspector O'Connell. We had a nice little chat. So friendly that one." She rolled her eyes as Alex let out a small laugh. "He let me have first dibs on you. Ethan is here too, and they too had a nice little chat. Apparently he's willing to strike a deal with DOJ and give them what they need to bring down Estavez."

"That doesn't sound so bad. What about Jack—any news?"

Sydney sighed and pushed her long blond hair over her shoulder. "No. No news of him yet."

"How does that make you feel?" His face softened as he looked at her.

She shrugged. That was the part where she felt conflicted. When she first found out Jack was alive, she was furious, indignant. The news brought about so much fury and pain, she just wanted him to go back to being dead. It was like reliving his death all over again. But when they caught up to him on the path and he reacted the way he did toward Ethan, wanting to protect her, her feelings changed.

Jack kept saying over and over again he had a plan that included her.

"I don't know…"

Alex reached over and squeezed her hand. "You deserve better, Sydney."

She knew he was right. Sydney looked down at him. His head was heavily bandaged, but he still managed to look ruggedly handsome. She leaned down and kissed him on the lips. Alex reached up and placed his hand on her cheek as they lingered for a moment, lips locked in place. She felt electricity course through her body, awakening something within her that she had kept buried.

Sydney heard the click of the door handle and pulled back. Inspector O'Connell made a loud entrance into the room. Not only did his wide girth seem to fill the room, his presence seemed to overshadow anything else the light touched. Sydney leaned back, away from Alex, as if being caught kissing a middle school boyfriend.

"Alex, glad to have you back with us," O'Connell said, making a direct path toward him. He reached down and shook his hand firmly. Sydney guessed that was as warm and friendly as the inspector got.

"Sydney," he said, nodding in her direction. "Might I have a few words with Alex?"

"Sure," she said. She leaned down and gave Alex a quick kiss on the cheek. "Don't be a stranger."

O'Connell raised an eyebrow at her as she walked out of the room. She breezed down the hospital hallway, a bit lighter on her feet than when she had entered. As she pulled out her phone to call an Uber, she thought about what that kiss meant. Maybe there was more there between them or maybe not. But after everything Alex had done for her, the kiss was well deserved.

A few minutes later Sydney was ducking into a silver four-door sedan with an Uber sticker on the front. She was ready to get to the airport, join Marissa, and leave Jamaica behind for good. The driver was wearing a Chicago Cubs baseball cap. Sydney noticed it as she stepped into the car.

Sydney caught up on emails and direct messages as they drove. When they were about five minutes from the airport, she finally spoke to the driver.

"Are you a Cubs fan?" she asked politely.

"I used to be," he said, looking in the rearview mirror. When she caught a glimpse of his brown eyes, her heartbeat froze in her chest.

"Jack? What the hell are you doing here?"

"Don't worry, Sydney. I just wanted to say goodbye."

"Goodbye? Where are you going?"

"I don't know yet, but I need a fresh start." He flicked his turn signal on and they made a right turn into a large airport terminal. "I'm sure you need one too."

Sydney sat in silence, too stunned to speak. There were so many words that she could have said, feelings she could have shared. But it didn't matter now; she had changed. Jack didn't hold the same meaning in her heart anymore.

As Jack stopped her in front of the private terminal, he jumped out of the car. He ran around the side and pulled the door open for her. She could smell the heat from the concrete drive mixed with his oaky, cinnamon scent. She had always loved the way he smelled.

As he peered up at her from under his baseball cap, he said, "I'm sorry Sydney, for everything." He touched her arm lightly as he spoke.

"I know," said Sydney, remaining perfectly still. "I... forgive you." She pulled her vintage bag a little tighter to her body as she moved toward the airport hangar. She could almost see a faint sheen of tears over his eyes, but he said nothing.

"Goodbye, Jack."

"Goodbye," he said.

And with that, Sydney turned her back and walked toward the private jet waiting for her.

FORTY-FOUR
SYDNEY

SYDNEY LEANED back into the caramel leather seat next to the jet window and tried to get comfortable. She should have been comfortable; the seats were probably filled with down. She ran her hand down the arm rest, watching as the long airplane hangars zoomed past her, occasionally punctuated by a cluster of palm trees. She was finally leaving Jamaica behind. She had only been there a few days—less than a week total—but it had seemed like an eternity given the epic events that had transpired during her stay.

In many ways she was a different Sydney than the one who had left Chicago last week. She didn't need an Ambien; she needed clarity. She felt stronger and more sure of herself in some ways, in others she felt exhausted and jaded.

As the palm trees grew small on the ground beneath her, she thought about her next steps.

She still loved fashion, as was evidenced by the hour she spent getting ready this morning, curling her hair, splashing on her makeup, and pulling on her favorite cashmere sweater. She had even managed to post a photo on her site, which felt superficial and decidedly fake. But the reality was, she still had bills to pay and she couldn't just throw all the work from the last few years out the window. But she knew she couldn't go back to that perfect life she had portrayed. She wanted something real. She thought about writing a book, telling her experience as an average girl who was wrestled into the workings of an international criminal.

"Champagne?" she heard Marissa say as she walked into the main cabin.

"Yes, thanks," she said.

Marissa placed two fluted glasses on the table between them and began to pour. As she sat down across from her, Sydney smiled.

"So, I guess Jack and Ethan turned out to be different from who we thought they were," Sydney said as she tipped her glass back into her mouth. Marissa sighed.

"I knew Ethan was a bit of a bad boy. I guess that was a part of him I was attracted to." She looked out the window. "But I had no idea how bad he really was. I guess I have a lot to learn about people."

"You're telling me. I thought I had the perfect life. I was so focused on impressing a bunch of people I didn't even know, I missed all the lies that were piling up around me."

Marissa looked at her. "Don't be so hard on yourself, Syd."

Sydney smiled. "I wish Lizzy was here."

"Me too," she said, cocking her head as her eyes welled up with tears. Marissa held up her glass in the sunlight that was peering through the windows. "To Lizzy."

"To Lizzy," Sydney responded, tipping her glass to meet Marissa's. "And to the truth."

A LETTER FROM LEAH

Thank you for reading *What Lies in Paradise.* I hope you enjoyed it. If you'd like to keep up-to-date with my latest releases, just sign up here and I'll let you know when my next novel comes out:

WWW.LEAHCUPPS.COM

I'm also thrilled to get feedback about my books, so if you enjoyed it, I would love if you could post a short review online or tell your friends about it. Your opinion makes a huge difference helping people discover my books for the first time.

I love chatting with readers, so please feel free to get in touch via my facebook page, through GoodReads or my website.

Thanks so much!

Leah Cupps

Lightning Source UK Ltd.
Milton Keynes UK
UKHW020604070120
356492UK00006B/142/P

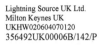

9 781734 405507